Physician Suicide Letters

Answered by Pamela Wible, M.D.

Dedicated to all medical students,
to every child who has ever dreamed of being a doctor,
and to all those who have lost their lives in pursuit of healing others.

Physician Suicide Letters

Answered by Pamela Wible, M.D.

Pamela Wible, M.D., Publishing
Oregon

Table of Contents

Introduction

Despite it all, I remain an optimist.

Medical school knocked me to my knees. I haven't been the same since. Even though I still have a sparkle in my eyes and joy in my heart, a piece of me is missing. I can never get it back. I've tried. My innocence is gone.

Like most students, I just wanted to help people. I wanted to heal the broken world, the injured hearts and souls of patients who would one day entrust me with their lives. Instead, I nearly lost my own life. The memorization-regurgitation method of medical education disturbed my creative, non-linear mind. I studied constantly—spitting back medical minutiae for multiple-choice tests. I'm an average test-taker, though I excel with patients. I'm happiest helping people.

But it's difficult to be happy (or help people) in a medical culture that condones hazing, bullying, sexual harassment, and teaching by public humiliation. In my school, there seemed to be no end to the filthy jokes that demeaned female patients and classmates. In lectures, my instructors actually made fun of vegetarians for eating "health food." When I protested the dog labs, where first-year medical students had to kill dogs, the dean diagnosed me with "Bambi Syndrome." I was belittled because I cared—about animals, about people, about my own health, and about this planet we call home.

I cried my way through the first year of medical school. As long as my tears kept flowing, I knew I would be okay. Crying meant that I could still feel pain. If I stopped crying, I thought I would go numb. One night I cried so much that I awoke the next day with my eyelids swollen shut. I could no longer bear to see the brutality.

I survived by clinging to my dream of being a caring family physician, of making house calls, of being a trusted and loving neighborhood doctor. I graduated from med school, completed residency, and got a job. I hated it. So I moved to another clinic. Then another. And another. After a decade of seven-minute visits at assembly-line clinics, I was nothing more than a factory worker. I felt like my dream was dead.

I wanted to die.

And, I thought I was the only doctor who felt this way.

Then I got a crazy idea. What if I asked for help? Not from the profession that wounded me. Instead I asked patients: "What is ideal health care? What kind of doctor do you want?"

They told me that an ideal doctor is happy, has a big heart and a great love for people and service. They described an ideal clinic as a sanctuary, a safe place, a place of wisdom with fun flannel gowns and complimentary massage while waiting, where nobody is turned away for lack of money.

I followed their instructions and opened *their* ideal clinic—the first clinic designed entirely by patients!

I started writing and speaking about my dream-come-true clinic, how I survived med school, and how I recovered from my occupationally induced depression and suicidal thoughts.

Then something weird and unexpected happened. I started getting letters from suicidal medical students and doctors. I wasn't the only one who had felt this way!

Each year more than one million Americans lose their doctors to suicide, and nobody ever tells patients the truth—the real reason they can't see their doctors ever again.

Nobody talks about our doctors jumping from hospital rooftops, overdosing in call rooms, hanging themselves in hospital chapels. It's medicine's dirty secret—and it's covered up by our hospitals, clinics, and medical schools.

No medical school wants to be known as the "Suicide School." No hospital wants to be #1 for interns jumping from rooftops. No student wants to become a doctor in order to kill themselves. It's the ultimate oxymoron: the barefoot shoemaker, the starving chef, the suicidal doctor.

So what the hell is going on? Why is the plague of physician and medical student suicide such a secret? Why am I the one piecing this together? I'm a solo family doc, yet somehow I've become an investigative reporter, a special-ist in physician suicide. Why? Mostly because I can't stop asking why. Why did both doctors I dated in med school die by suicide? Why did eight doctors kill themselves—just in my sweet little Oregon town?

There are answers. Finding them requires being willing to look at some very disturbing facts. It also requires the willingness to engage with people who have experienced and who continue to experience a great deal of pain. So I keep talking and writing—and listening for the truth. And because I'm listening with my heart and soul 24/7, my cell phone has turned into a suicide hotline and I've received hundreds of letters from suicidal physicians all over the world.

You may be wondering why so many people who want to help people end up killing themselves. That's why I wrote this book.

A Message to Medical Students & Doctors

If I could tell medical students and my fellow doctors one thing, it would be this:

You are not alone. You are not defective. Our profession is. Medicine has lost its way. By claiming your true calling as a healer, you can prevent future tragedies. It's up to each of us. We can reach out to our brothers and sisters in medicine and help one another—now. Every medical student and physician should have access to this life-saving information. Please share this book. If you are a family member of a medical student or physician, I hope these letters give you much-needed insight and a new level of empathy for your loved one who might be struggling silently.

A Message to Patients

Why should you care about the impact of our dysfunctional medical system on your doctor's health?

Because it affects you. You may lose your own doctor to suicide. But even if that doesn't happen, you may be receiving poor care because your doctor is depressed or suicidal. You may be wondering why your doctor does not seem to care. We start out caring and compassionate. Yet as doctors-in-training we are routinely hazed and bullied. Abused medical students become abused doctors, who may one day abuse patients. Ultimately, this cycle of abuse affects us all. *Physician Suicide Letters—Answered* takes you behind the white coat to reveal what really goes on inside your doctor and then empowers you to help stop the cycle of abuse so you can get the care you deserve.

Author's Note

This book includes real suicide letters—the last words of medical students and doctors. Also included are letters from surviving family members, colleagues, and patients. Most letters are from suicidal physicians seeking my help. All have been published with permission. A few have been edited for clarity. Some names have been changed upon request to safeguard the careers of those who have written to me.

Physician Suicide Letters—Answered inspired my TEDMED talk on physician suicide, in which I read excerpts from letters in this book. Several chapters reference my articles and videos on physician suicide. These can be found in Resources at the end of the book.

All proceeds from this book will be used to humanize our medical education system and help save the lives of suicidal medical students and doctors.

Disclaimer

I'm not a psychiatrist and have no formal training in suicide prevention. Yet a number of medical students and physicians have told me that I helped to save their lives. How? By listening. By caring. By sharing my experiences and the experiences of others. My hope is that these stories will continue to help others find validation and inspiration to live.

Chapter letters and referenced articles are for general information only. I'm your friend. I'm not your doctor (unless you are one of my patients in Oregon). Each person is unique. Please contact a medical professional to discuss your specific condition. If you are a medical student or doctor struggling now, please see "Our message of hope for medical students & doctors" in Resources. If you are actively suicidal, please call your physician or go to your local emergency room.

Part One
The Problem

I

Post Traumatic
Student Disorder

Post traumatic student disorder is a normal reaction
to a traumatic educational experience.

1

Anna

January 25, 2015

Dear Pamela,

Thank you so much for the truths you speak for so many. Many times in my years of medicine I have said to trusted friends and to several therapists, "Something happened to me in med school."

I was happy, secure, and mostly unafraid until med school. I recall in vivid detail the first orientation day. Our anatomy professor stood before an auditorium filled with 125 eager, nervous, idealistic would-be healers and said these words: "If you decide to commit suicide, do it right so you do not become a burden to society." He then described in anatomical detail how to commit suicide.

I have often wondered how many auditoriums full of new students heard those words from him. I am sure someone stood in front of us and told us what a wonderful and rewarding profession we had chosen. I do not remember those words. But I do remember how to successfully commit suicide— with a gun.

One month later, on the eve of our first monthly round of six exams in one day, I had my first full-blown panic attack. I had no idea what was happening. I thought I was losing my mind. I took a leave of absence and made up excuses. I returned untreated with maladaptive compulsive behavior, completed med school, survived the public "pimp sessions," and all the rest.

[Pimping is a "teaching" technique in which a student is grilled with rapid-fire questions (often about obscure medical minutiae). These much-feared public interrogation sessions can be so malicious that the student may be left crying—in front of peers, staff, and patients.]

No one ever suggested that the process was brutal, or the responsibility frightening, and no one offered us help. I have maintained contact with only one colleague from med school, so I do not know how the others fared.

Through the many years of training, and through what would appear to the observer a successful career in a surgical subspecialty and now into retirement, I have carried the anxiety, and the depression, and the fear. Perhaps entirely unrelated to those first days in med school, but still something happened to me, and probably to many of us, that changed us forever. I still remember how to successfully commit suicide, because someone who had power over me at a vulnerable time described the details. And we wonder why . . .

Anna

* * *

January 25, 2015

Dear Anna,

I can't stop crying after reading your letter. Sadly, there have been other auditoriums and other professors who gave the same lecture. Another physician wrote, "An anatomy professor did inform us that we would commit suicide at a higher than average rate and told us from the lectern how to accomplish it successfully. I considered following the instructions on three occasions: once in my third year, once as an intern, and most recently when my four-year-old patient died." So Anna, you are not alone.

Pamela

* * *

January 25, 2015

Pamela,

First, every word I wrote is true and there is so much more (much of it un-believable gender-based harassment, but that is a different issue entirely). And it took me a long time to stop crying quietly to myself. My husband is a general contractor and really has no idea what is wrong with me. I could never explain it to him.

Please know that I am not in danger of suicide (I have a mother, a daughter, and a grandson who would be devastated, so that is not currently an issue).

How in the world can you do everything you are doing to support physicians while practicing family medicine?

As I read and thought about your wonderful posts and response to my email, I thought it is possible that this is the best healing I have found in thirty-five years. Thank you for speaking and writing about what has been the truth for so many of us who have been afraid to talk about it.

Anna

* * *

January 25, 2015

Anna,

How in the world can I help suicidal physicians while practicing family med-icine with no staff? Great question. I'm super-organized and I ask for help. A funny thing happens when you ask for help—people want to help you! My patients and community sustain me with food, love, money (I've never sent anyone to collections!). One patient even makes my clothes! Plus I've got my own personal team of healers who keep me well. I get weekly massage, coaching, exercise. I drink green smoothies, sing gospel music while hiking through the woods, and pet my cat a lot. :)

Pamela

* * *

June 8, 2015

Hi Pamela,

I am doing surprisingly well. Since I contacted you, I decided that I really needed to take the bull (my life) by the horns and have done several very active things (connected with a wonderful online support group, got serious about yoga, started setting limits at home, etc.). Thank you again for the work you do. I really think that connecting with you has helped me to realize *it is not just me! There is nothing really wrong with me!* We have been traumatized!

Anna

2

Maria

June 14, 2013

Dear Dr. Wible,

I definitely graduated from med school with PTSD. It has changed me forever. My mom's friend, someone that I have known since I was born, saw me for the first time since I went to med school and she said to my mom, "She has changed so much. Was it worth it?" I wish I could change back, but I realize that I will never be the same again.

We had two suicides and one murder, skull crushed with a bat, and one serving life in prison for murdering a classmate during a delusional episode after not sleeping for a month. Yes, I went to a hard-core school. PTSD isn't benign. It truly affects you to the core. It changes your brain. It makes you numb and it makes you have a terrible memory. I used to have an amazing memory.

Please change medical education. We were so beaten down on our clinical rotations. I almost dropped out after the first week of my first rotation in surgery. Literally I had the papers ready. It takes a lot for me to break down and cry, but I think I cried at least once a week on that rotation (twelve weeks of hell) along with everyone else. But we hid it from each other, of course.

I hope you continue to help physicians like you are doing. Even having access to something to read like your blog helps tremendously. It makes me feel as if I am not so alone. I know that there are others in the same boat. We don't always need much, just something every so often to keep things going. Thank you so much for being such an awesome role model. I hope one day I can be the same.

Maria

* * *

June 14, 2013

Maria,

Your med school sounds barbaric. I'd love to talk to you. Hey, how did you find me? We should meet one day soon. Do you ever get out to Oregon? If so, you gotta come to our physician retreat!

Pamela

* * *

June 14, 2013

Dr. Wible,

How exactly does this retreat change things for the physicians who attend? Have some stated that they no longer wished to end their lives because of the few days there? I am just curious as it seems to be quite powerful.

Maria

* * *

June 14, 2013

Hey Maria,

Yes. Doctors claim that the retreat has helped to save their lives. Kind of a love bath mixed with amazing practice management tools. It's hard to explain. Hey, call me anytime. Come for free! I'm here for ya, babe!

Pamela

* * *

June 15, 2013

Hey Wible,

I greatly appreciate your invitation. I am not able to come. Believe me. I would love to, but I wanted to tell you thanks for even asking. It truly does make a difference.

Things have been rough lately. My anatomy professor just committed suicide recently. I understand his pain. I would be indebted to you if you could add me to your mailing list, updates, or whatever you have set up. Your site has helped me. And please don't become jaded. Please help the next generation of docs. We work so hard to get to a place where we can actually finally help people. The road sometimes can be hell, sometimes it is just rough, sometimes it is cake or so they act like it is cake. Sometimes it is difficult. Sometimes it is worse than difficult. But I went for it because I can't imagine a life without medicine. I love it. It is what I know. It is what I have experienced. I am only medicine. Nothing else.

Thanks for being something for me to read at the very worst of times. And if you ever want to send me something that might help, articles etc., that would be awesome!

Maria

* * *

December 6, 2013

Wible,

Thanks for calling me back. Sorry I needed to talk so long on your birthday. I'm okay now. Happy holidays!

Maria

* * *

June 7, 2014

Wible,

Am having a really tough night tonight. Really just hard sometimes for me but I am happy to know that there is someone out there interested in the world, in the pain that medicine sometimes is. Rough week, lots of deaths in people less than forty.

Maria

3

Lisa

November 3, 2014

Hello Dr. Wible,

I'm a surgery resident in New York. I began my residency in California and during that time was very depressed due to abuse within my training program. My depression impacted my performance and I was eventually fired. I was lucky enough to find another position and continue my training. However, some days I feel my depression and despair returning—primarily when I feel my career has been irreparably damaged by my departure from my first residency program. Those feelings were initially tied to hazing and bullying that are an integral part of the educational program there. Sometimes I can still hear those attendings [senior physicians] in my head saying things like "Watching you operate is like watching a retarded monkey" or "Do they even teach anatomy at your medical school? Our students know more than you!" It's paralyzing. I am reaching out to you for two reasons: I'm interested in eradicating the abuse in medical education. I'd like to have a career in academics and to influence policy regarding the treatment of trainees. More importantly, can you help me make the flashbacks stop? Can you help me not worry so much about my future? Can you help me with my depression related to my change in career trajectory? Thank you for your work!

Lisa

* * *

November 3, 2014

Dear Lisa,

Yes! We need kind-hearted teachers and great mentors in medicine, not bitter cynics. I'd love to help med schools humanize their curricula. There is so much that can be done to change medical culture so we can stop the needless suffering inflicted upon students.

Not exactly sure how to stop flashbacks, a symptom of PTSD. Are you in counseling? I recommend all medical students and doctors get weekly counseling and massage. Physicians who fear repercussions tell me they choose to go "off the grid" so they don't have to worry about "reporting" it. You deserve care and love and support too! How can we care for patients if we don't get the care we need? Sadly, it's unlikely that the Western medical system that injured you would be the source of your healing. Unless you are actively suicidal and need meds, I highly recommend that you seek a holistic health care team that can help you re-integrate your body-mind-spirit. Reductionist medicine (the foundation of Western medicine) is the opposite of holistic medicine. So it's no surprise that so many med students and physicians suffer from mind-body-spirit *dis*integration. Make sense?

Pamela

* * *

November 30, 2014

Pamela,

Thanks so much for getting in touch with me. We need to talk openly about this abuse. Please feel free to share my letter if it can help others; however, change my name and delete the name of my school. When I left I had to sign a non-disclosure statement. Basically I'm not allowed to tell anyone how terribly I was treated there.

I've been meaning to get in touch with you. My close friend Jake committed suicide last month. No one knows why he chose to jump off a parking structure after his hospital shift on a Sunday night. He had been planning a Hawaiian vacation and sounded well when I spoke with him the week before. Jake had a history of depression and anxiety. It seemed as if the worst was behind him and he was coping much better. His death was a shock to everyone who knew him. We used to talk at least a few times a week; I miss him every day. Incidentally, Jake and I were pretty good friends with Greg [chapter 35].

Thank you again for thinking of me. Please keep doing the work that you do. It's an area that is too often ignored.

Lisa

4

Christian

March 12, 2013

Dear Pamela,

I'm a physician in the UK and things here appear to be the same [as in the US]. I have several colleagues who have committed suicide over the years, and I feel lucky to have survived myself. I am particularly disturbed by the prevalence of PTSD among colleagues. Yes indeed I was traumatized in medical school and it continues to happen, but we get accustomed to it—to the point of becoming an abused class.

Christian

* * *

March 13, 2013

Dear Christian,

I was hoping it would be better elsewhere. Very disheartening. I always tell docs, "You can't be a victim and a healer at the same time." Speaking the truth is the first step to healing. That so many caring young medical students graduate with PTSD is a crime against humanity. We pay more than $300,000 tuition for this abuse. What a racket!

Pamela

5

Patricia

March 23, 2015

Pamela,

I am not surprised at the number of suicides among medical practitioners. I was a nurse for years and went back to school to be a physician assistant. There is so much abuse handed out in training. At the time I was in school, we still had some thirty-six-hour shifts. It was difficult. At least at the university that I attended they had a buddy program. All of the first-year students were given a third-year student to help show us around and be a mentor. The problem was that before we even started our first classes, my mentor committed suicide. She was in her car on her way home still close to the hospital when she stopped at a red light then picked up a gun and shot herself in the head. The person behind her was a physician at the hospital. These things are not that unusual. It's a sad state of affairs.

Patricia

II

Anti-Mentors & Tormentors

Students describe medical school as an anti-mentorship program.
They meet a lot of doctors they'd never want to become.

6

Vicky

February 12, 2015

Pamela,

When I share what happens in our academic medical center with my non-medical friends, they are astonished and disbelieving. The level of bullying in my institution is amazing, including a faculty member seriously suggesting that a resident's mistake was so heinous that he should "off" himself. When I speak about changing the culture of medicine, my colleagues think it is impossible to support financially. In our institution, money is a deal breaker. We have a patient wellness program with financial/insurance premium incentives, but as far as I know, no physician wellness program with incentives. I will watch what happens with you with interest. Keep doing it.

Vicky

* * *

February 13, 2015

Vicky,

It's not costly or complicated to end bullying and hazing. It's been outlawed at elementary schools, fraternities, and pretty much everywhere—except health care. How much does it really cost to be kind and compassionate? How much does it cost to replace hundreds of doctors who off themselves?

Pamela

7

Alison

October 31, 2014

Dear Pamela,

I'm a GP (general practitioner) in the UK—it's not just in the US that these problems are occurring. I'm currently off sick with anxiety/depression—this is my third episode and I'm only thirty-one. The first episode started in medical school during a particularly unpleasant "teaching session" where I was ripped apart in front of a patient and my peers. My best friend stood next to me whispering, "It's okay, it's okay" in a bid to stop me from breaking down then and there. We moved to the next patient for one of my peers to be cross-examined, when this patient looked at me and offered me a tissue because she could see the tears in my eyes.

The second episode happened less than two years after medical school, although I'm surprised I lasted that long. The grueling nights on call instilled such fear in me that I would get diarrhea before each shift and at one point I actually considered making myself ill by breaking a leg, in a bid to get out of work. It didn't help that I felt responsible and blamed for the death of a patient and received no support.

Currently I just don't think I can continue with medicine—the job is wearing me down so much that I can't seem to notice the positives anymore. It's not helped that in the UK, GPs are currently being blamed for every problem in the NHS [National Health System] by politicians and the media. We are told we're lazy and overpaid and should do more for less money, etc. Patients have become self-entitled and abusive/aggressive, thinking that they know how to manage their illnesses better than us. We're just here to hand over the prescriptions they demand. I don't know how things can improve, to be honest.

Alison

* * *

November 1, 2014

Dear Alison,

Bullying doctors for sport and political gain. Terrible! Is there an organization in the UK that advocates for doctors, protects them from this abuse? We certainly need one in the US where we essentially have no labor law protection. We need to be less resilient and more resistant to abuse. Remember: you are not defective, the system is. Please take care of yourself.

Pamela

8

Maureen

April 5, 2014

Pamela,

As a physician who spent a year in residency avoiding walking next to busy streets, parking on the bottom of the garage, and refusing to have any medications in my house because I knew that I could, at any moment, use them as a means to escape, I thank you for your articles.

I recognize that it's hard for many non-physicians to "feel bad" for doctors—we are seen as privileged. Many of us are egotistical. All of us are fallible. And, like everyone else, all of us are capable of plummeting to the depths of hell quickly and of feeling like there is no escape.

What I don't think many non-physicians understand is some of the unique circumstances we face. Even other non-physician medical providers don't typically have the same experience.

Most of us have to work our hardest to be at the top in high school and to get into a good college, then in college to do well on the MCAT and get into a good medical school. Then in medical school to do well on shelf and board exams to get into the residency we want. Even then, there's no guarantee of that residency. We could work very hard for four years towards one specific goal and then be required to pursue a different specialty.

Once we're in residency, what feels like indentured servitude begins. We can't really choose where we go. We can list the places we'd be willing to go, and a computer decides for us. We can't negotiate our contracts. We are frequently seen and treated by patients, other medical personnel, and (worst) our attending [supervising] physicians as unwelcomed intruders. Attending physicians who feel that it's their right to treat residents like scum exist, and if you are unlucky enough to have one choose you as his/her pet destruction project, you have just bought into three to seven years of abject torture from someone who can literally end your entire career in a moment.

After residency, physicians work hard for their patients. We bring them home with us, figuratively speaking, every night. We work endless hours and sacrifice our families to help someone else's family member. Sometimes we're rewarded with the knowledge that we did our very best for someone, sometimes we find people who are grateful for our help. All too often, and more frequently these days, we find people who declare us slaves to pharmaceutical companies or the government. They declare that they know more than any doctor because they've read something on the Internet. They rant on about how doctors only want to make money and don't care about patients, and they respond to articles about the problem of physician suicide with comments like "I don't feel sorry for doctors at all."

This doctor is working hard to pay off student debt that amounts to a very nice house. I really do love my patients and I do my best for them. I feel better most days, but I would never recommend medical school to another human being because one simply never comes out the same. Your writing helps us realize we're not alone, even if non-physician members of society are likely to think we get what we deserve.

Maureen

9

Glenn

November 21, 2014

Dear Pamela,

Thanks for your fine work. It's nice to see such a serious problem discussed openly. I attended Harvard Medical School, made what the books assured me was a reliable suicide attempt, woke up thirty-six hours later. Blind luck. I was offered an antidepressant, time off doing research, and the choice to return or not. Nothing more. Studying was no big deal: that was like asking a fish to swim. Sleep deprivation was devastating, and I have come to see it as completely counterproductive as an educational strategy. It risks countless patients' lives and serves only as an advanced form of hazing, more thorough and relentless and of greater duration than any hazing I've found elsewhere. Other forms of bullying take on new toxicity when one is so weakened and vulnerable. So I got out. I'm a nurse and a teacher now. People often ask me "why" I'm not a doctor. Why? Because I stood up for myself, at long last.

Glenn

* * *

December 4, 2014

Glenn,

Good for you. First do no harm to yourself. So sorry that our medical "education" system continues to torment so many beautiful, young people who just want to help people. Public outrage is mounting. Neither patients nor physicians will tolerate this abuse much longer. The truth shall set us free.

Pamela

10

Sarah

November 3, 2014

Dr. Wible,

I was dismissed from medical school in the beginning of my fourth year because I had a medical condition that didn't help the school's "technical standards." I suffered abuse my entire third year from residents and physicians telling me that I wasn't fit to be in medicine, that if I knew what was good for me I would just drop out. My school told me that being sick was akin to being unprofessional, and that I should give up my dreams of wanting to become a physician. They pulled me into their administrative office several times to harass me, and eventually told me that I was dismissed. I couldn't think, I couldn't breathe. If I hadn't called my parents immediately and spoken to them, I don't know what I would have done because only the worst was running through my head at that time. Medical schools need to be more attuned to their students' needs and psyches before treating them like slaves or robots with no regard for human emotion.

Sarah

* * *

November 3, 2014

Sarah,

Your medical school kicked you out due to a physical illness? How cruel. That's gotta be illegal. The Americans with Disabilities Act protects against discrimination based on mental and physical illnesses. Don't let them get away with that. Don't give up your future as a healer. [I asked Sarah to explain the "technical standards." She responded, "Sorry, legally not allowed to discuss." Victims are often forced to sign non-disclosure agreements to keep quiet about the abuse.]

Pamela

* * *

January 23, 2015

Pamela,

I received your package today. A slurry of emotions rose up as I realized I am embarking on a wonderful journey towards change and hope. I was especially touched by your handwritten note and the handout from your lecture. I'd also like to mention that there is confetti all over my desk—and I love it! Looking forward to living my dream in medicine! I won't give up on my goal of helping children!

Sarah

11

Vincent

August 25, 1998

I love you mom. I'm so sorry.

Vincent

* * *

September 17, 2014

Hi Dr. Wible,

My son Vincent was into his second month of residency when we lost him. He was twenty-five years old.

He chose the inner-city hospital believing that it could offer him the best training in surgery. He was excited to get started but somehow was apprehensive knowing that he would now be on his own and lives of patients would totally depend on him. Nonetheless, he was ready to give it his best.

It was apparent that he became more and more disappointed and disillusioned as the days passed. He had an apartment close to the hospital, but he would drive forty-five minutes to come home at every brief chance he had from the long and sleepless days and nights in the hospital just to stay in his room and sleep. He had no appetite, the laughs and jokes were gone, and he lost a lot of weight. While we were concerned, we thought it was just part of the adjustment to this hectic and demanding profession.

After a month I asked him if he ever got paid. Being a mother, I was excited for him to get his first paycheck no matter how small it was. He said that he had to go to this other building to pick up the check during office hours and just did not have the chance but would certainly try in the few next days. He came home one day and told me that while they were in the operating room for hours waiting for something (he was not doing anything), he had asked his senior attending physician if he could run out to pick up his check. He said that the attending physician got very annoyed at him in front of the whole staff. Needless to say, he felt very embarrassed and stupid, not to mention that Vincent was a very sensitive person. I can still picture his sad face while telling me the incident. The horrible guilt I had of causing him that unnecessary shame will stay with me forever.

One time he was talking about closing up on a surgery (he prided himself in doing beautiful suture work and gently catching an infant at birth) and feeling good at what he was doing but he was told to hurry up and just wrap it up. I thought that was funny, but he took that seriously. He said he was aware of the importance of not taking too long—just wanted to do a good job. He talked about his doubts about saving this one guy who jumped out of a building when he was caught raping a young girl who was also being treated in an adjacent room. [Surgery residents are often inserted into crime scenes where they are treating perpetrators and victims. With no emotional support or sleep!]

Just once he had a pleasant story during all these hospital days: There were two nurse assistants who were very nice to him. He said that they told him to make sure to tell them if anyone gave him a hard time and they would take care of them. One time, he brought home a bag of banana chips these two ladies gave him. He knew I liked them and wanted to share them with me. He certainly appreciated and needed that little act of kindness that was so sparingly given while struggling to sort out his troubling emotions, disappointments, and disillusions. And he kept these all to himself. There was no one who would listen or understand. They were all too busy. There was no place or time for emotions. He just needed to please everyone at any cost. He was trapped in this hospital darkness with no hope for a better tomorrow.

It has been sixteen years since he passed away but it feels like he was here just yesterday. I kept wondering why no one helped him. How did I miss all the signs? Somehow, he must have been wanting to reach out but was too proud to admit to what would be viewed as a failure. God forbid, doctors cannot be losers. He was a very dear son to me and I believe with love and faith that he is now in a better and peaceful place and endures no pain or sadness. He may not be here physically, but his spirit is so real and stays on with me every minute and up to when we meet again.

My biggest regret, and something that does not slip my mind even for a day, is that I—the mother and probably the closest to him—did not pay attention to the obvious signs that Vincent exhibited weeks before that horrible day. Things could have possibly been different. Vincent was so alone.

I thank you again for your time and dedication to maybe bring about awareness to this disturbing situation that harms our young doctors. Please let me know if there is anything I can do to help.

Warm regards,
Aida

* * *

September 6, 2014

Dear Dr. Wible,

My family had our share of personal tragedy when we lost our nephew while on his seventh week of surgery residency in his dream program at one of New York's prestigious surgery programs.

He was the oldest among the children in the family, a vibrant, happy person who sailed through undergraduate school and obtained his first choice in the match program. We were all ecstatic when he started his residency at twenty-five; he was the family clown and everyone was so proud of his personal achievements—until that fateful day we heard from his landlord the tragic news. We were all stunned and could not believe he was really gone.

There were no signs of depression. We knew he was tired and sleep deprived. He told stories of how he and his partner in rotation fell asleep leaning against the walls while waiting for their patient's turn for a scan. He spoke of them as funny tales of residency. He spoke of how sisters, victims of a car accident brought into the emergency room, stunned him for a moment because they reminded him of his mother and me who often travel together without seatbelts. In hindsight, they were tales of disaster looming in the horizon. We had no idea how the combination of sleep deprivation, hospital experiences, and life-and-death responsibilities were affecting him. As we learned later, these are common elements that affect these young doctors in the most devastating way!

In his memory, and to keep his dreams to serve alive, the family established foundations in two medical schools. Both are intended to provide mental health support: one in a workshop format, the other as a lecture series provided by psychiatrists to first-year residents. Our hope is that these foundations will continue in perpetuity to remind young residents that there is help, someone to call during those first critical months of residency. These young doctors who just moved to their programs in a new city, with no family or support system, are overwhelmed with their expanded responsibilities while putting in 80+ hours of work a week. How can we allow someone making life-and-death decisions less sleep than the average worker? These work schedules for interns are inhumane!

Edna

* * *

October 22, 2015

Dear Aida & Edna,

I have been invited to give a TEDMED talk on physician suicide to 850 leaders in health and medicine—plus the talk will be transmitted livestream to medical schools and hospitals in hundreds of countries. These talks can get millions of views online and be translated into dozens of languages. I would love to share Vincent's story and his photo. Please let me know if that is okay with you. The surgeon general will be there as will many important people who can help change the medical system so we can stop the abuse of our young doctors.

In gratitude,
Pamela

* * *

November 2, 2015

Hi Dr. Wible,

Thank you so much for the update on your presentation. While viewing anything related to Vincent remains as painful as always, I appreciate that you considered him to be a part of your sincere intentions to eliminate or at least minimize these sad and tragic happenings and waste of young lives. Congratulations and good luck in your endless efforts to make a difference. Please let me know if there is anything at all my family and I can do to support this huge and challenging endeavor. God bless you.

Aida

* * *

November 30, 2015

Dear Pamela,

Aida shared the news clip and your photo taken at TEDMED. You are doing a wonderful job carrying the message and purpose of our efforts to bring awareness of physician suicides to the medical community. Thank you from the bottom of our hearts! We hope that the tides will turn and the awareness you bring will prevent future heartaches for the families and lost potential for the bright, hardworking, dedicated and maybe sometimes idealistic, inexperienced young doctors. May the Force be with you always!

Edna

12

Shelley

April 21, 2015

Pamela,

I need help.

I need a residency in Los Angeles. It will save my life. If I had known that I would lose everything I had, including my identity, I would never have gone to medical school. Before I die, people need to know what happened to me, and hopefully there will be some safeguards put in place so these things can never again happen to any resident or student. Just left to die in a pile of student loans, watching the rest of the world carry on, just left here to die. How cruel we physicians are to each other. How can we be so cruel?

The training system encourages the production of the same type of cold-hearted physician. The one who grew up in higher socioeconomic status and lacks true empathy for poverty and mental illness. The lack of tolerance for any kind of delay or temporary withdrawal from training is a reflection of not only a traditionally male-dominated profession but also a traditionally higher socioeconomic status of the majority of the profession. Sometimes people have to resign temporarily; this is nothing new for anyone who has ever made it out of the cycle of poverty, especially the single mom. You just get it together and pick yourself up and try again. That's just part of the struggle for any strong person who made it out of the ghetto. You keep going; you may have to stop and take care of other problems, like food, clothing, shelter, transportation, childcare problems, but you fix those and then you keep going. Medical training has no tolerance for this and everyone knows it. That is why we keep producing the same type of doctors. There is no tolerance for the struggles of those less fortunate or for struggles typical of women with children.

I am also a nurse and my patients loved me as a doctor. They told me I was different in a way that they liked. Yet I was bullied out of the profession. My approach was comprehensive and thorough, and I never made the mistakes my colleagues made. I was going to be really good at it. But instead I was bullied out of it. It's beyond profoundly tragic. Words cannot describe my psychological pain. It's indescribable.

Shelley

* * *

April 21, 2015

Dear Shelley,

Don't give up! Tell your story and maybe I can help you publish it. Of course, I recommend that you get help and not suffer alone and do not let this profession take away your life. You are too precious to end your life and let the bullies win. All students should be safe from harassment and bullying in residency!

Pamela

* * *

April 21, 2015

Thank you Pamela,

That's a great idea to write my story. I'm just afraid of the backlash from the mean and abusive misogynists out there, ready to attack my perspective and blame me for resigning. I am very fearful of public humiliation now, since having had that experience. But I will do it anyway. It needs to be told. Too many people, even the medical boards who apparently are not even physicians anymore, are unaware of the abuses in medicine! The woman reviewing my application at the medical board mocked me when I said I was bullied. "The bullies?" she said. And I could hear the condescending smirk, like she wanted to laugh at me for mentioning bullying as if it was something for children.

Shelley

* * *

November 30, 2015

Pamela,

I am so sorry I have not written my story yet. I am still battling it out with the medical board and waiting for my free-and-clear license! The medical board is so incredibly ignorant. It's like they never heard of the concept of workplace bullying. After this, I think I would like to try to pass legislation that would prevent the board from denying a license without any evidence of patient harm. They are not even doctors! They went through every single evaluation written and passed judgment. I am so happy you are writing this book. You can use anything I wrote. I need to write my story.

Shelley

III

Death by Debt

Before the white coat ceremony, always fit the economic noose
tightly around each student's neck.

13

Kulthum

November 21, 2015

Hi Pamela,

I'm a fourth-year med student in a below-average school on the East coast. I performed well throughout medical school (top 20%), and have above-average board scores. I've applied for residency positions in three different fields. Unfortunately, I'm not getting interviews like I thought I would. I was advised that my application is rock solid; in fact, competitive. Doesn't seem to be the case given no interviews. I'm in significant debt (about $350,000), and though this is nothing foreign to med students, I come from a poor family and I would need to secure a residency to pay this back.

Now here's the thing. I don't anticipate matching into a residency program and I've made the decision to possibly end it all once I don't match. I have worked hard all my life. I did everything to get into the fields I've applied for (two of which are not even very competitive at all). Nothing has ever gone my way before or since starting medical school. I have gotten to this point after pushing through one struggle after another. During med school I had many significant tragedies in my family (deaths, illness, financial issues, to name a few). I fought through them. But I had to be cold to do it. I had to act like I did not care. I can't keep doing that to my family. I changed careers to go to med school. I pushed them into debt that never existed before school. Now I am facing the possibility of having an MD with no job in about seven months.

There is so much more to this. But I have hit on the important bits here. Thanks, Pam, for doing so much for the world with your blog. Thanks for giving me a forum to voice my thoughts. Bye.

Kulthum

* * *

December 3, 2015

Dear Kulthum,

Beyond infuriating that med schools leave qualified graduates unemployable! The public has no idea that there are not enough residency slots for graduates. It isn't commonly understood that without a residency *we can't work.* Patients are desperate for care and all these doctors like you want to care for them. Now more med schools are opening—all willing to take your money with no guarantee of employment!

Thankfully, there is hope for change on the horizon! In Missouri they passed legislation to allow a physician who graduates from medical school, and passes Step One and Step Two of the boards, but who has not completed a residency, to practice under a collaborative agreement with a licensed physician. This essentially mirrors the collaborative practice arrangement that has been in use in Missouri for many years relating to nurse practitioners.

Kulthum, you are not alone in this predicament. Please don't end your life. Promise you will at least call me. I have so many ideas for you. Seriously. It's not worth losing your life.

Pamela

* * *

December 3, 2015

Pamela,

I appreciate that you understand my predicament. I'm personally very concerned. I'm still going to try and match; but I know what I plan to do in the event that I don't match into a residency. I can't go past graduation with over $350,000 in debt (I've made all those around me, my family, enter a difficult spot by choosing to do this). Death will equal no debt, ultimately.

Kulthum

14

Dylan

June 19, 2014

Dear Pamela,

The decision to go to medical school was wrong. The idea that I could use the talents I have been blessed with to make a difference was a sham. I am called obscene names on satisfaction surveys by patients for not filling their prescriptions for narcotics/tranquilizers/amphetamines; called to task by supervisors for my arrogance at adhering to medical standards of care; and drowning in debt I can't escape by bankruptcy. I am in the process of stacking my life insurance to adequately care for my wife and children. I know how and where. Knowing I am not alone does not change things.

Dylan

* * *

June 19, 2014

Dylan,

I am here for you. I'd love to talk to you. Are you up?

Pamela

* * *

November 29, 2015

Dylan,

How are you? Are you okay? Please let me know that you are okay.

Pamela

* * *

November 30, 2015

Pamela,

I am struggling with the same issues and am still about where I was. Venting seems to help more than antidepressants. However the obscene reality of what physicians face simply to practice medicine cannot be discounted as a profoundly powerful contributing factor to the phenomenon of physician suicide. Like I said, venting helps, and I have been writing volumes on my laptop. Maybe I need to talk to your publisher.

Dylan

* * *

November 30, 2015

Dylan,

I am my publisher. Talk to me, babe. And keep writing. Writing the truth has been the best therapy for me.

Pamela

15

Michelle

June 27, 2013

Pamela,

I'm in my first year of practice and I can't begin to tell you how often I think of death. Not because I hate my life—I have a wonderful husband and family. But the pressures of daily life as a doctor are overwhelming. I work constantly! Even on my days off, I'm working. When I take a day off, I pay for it later by double the amount of work waiting for me. I have patients yelling at me when all I wanted to do was help. They try to fool me and manipulate me. Insurance companies deny my patients help—leaving me with no resources to help. My boss is a douche—unethical and dangerous. I want to build relationships and do what's right for my patients, but the company pushes me to see more and more patients in less and less time. I cry at work, I cry myself to sleep sometimes. I don't feel depressed, and I know my life has value, but sometimes the thought of suicide is just to escape the pressure of the profession. It's not like I can realistically give up the job, my calling. I'm neck deep in debt and will never be able to pay it back if I leave the profession.

Michelle

* * *

June 27, 2013

Hey Michelle,

Many physicians work in highly abusive and toxic medical practices, especially in primary care. Patients will fall to the level of dysfunction of the clinic. Dysfunctional clinic = dysfunctional patients. Misery loves company! Happy to help you off the assembly line. Open your own clinic. It's way easier than you think.

 Once you cut out the middlemen and no-value-added intermediaries, you can actually work less and earn more. Seriously. Don't let debt dictate your destiny and keep you trapped in a job you hate. And please don't give up your precious life. I'm here for you!

Pamela

IV

"Suck It Up"

Standard Treatment Plan

Suicidal Physician:
Suck it up.

Physician Suicide:
Sweep it under the rug.

16

Bobby

April 22, 2014

Dear Pamela,

I lost my grandpa, Bobby, in 1983. He was a family physician in a rural town in Southwest Alabama. For a period of time, he was the *only* doctor in said town. He had a previous attempt at suicide before he was successful. The first attempt was with an overdose, but my grandmother found him and he got the care he needed. What truly happened was swept under the rug, not only within our family, but in his circle of medical "friends." Unfortunately, despite him being "treated" by other colleagues, one of whom was a psychiatrist, he was told to essentially "suck it up." Sometime thereafter, he shot himself in the head sitting in the car outside the home my grandmother still lives in. Initially, as I stood in the shadow of my grandfather as a practicing family physician in the same town he practiced medicine in, I would wonder how such a well-loved and respected physician, husband, father, grandfather, and friend could get to the point where he no longer had the will to live. After having been in the profession as a practicing family physician for four years now, I get it.

Ashley

* * *

June 1, 2014

Ashley,

Thank you so much for writing about your grandfather. I am determined to prevent these physician suicides. I'd like to interview you and learn more about your grandfather's life and death. Wondering if you would be interested. You have such a compelling story. Have you ever felt suicidal? Would it be okay if I share your grandfather's story?

Pamela

* * *

June 1, 2014

Dear Pamela,

Absolutely. I'm humbled that you thought of my grandfather's story. To answer your question, yes and no, I have never felt suicidal but I have contemplated suicide (You may think these feelings are the same, but I think they are different degrees on a spectrum). I've never had a plan and know that I have a lot to live for, which makes me wonder just how bad it got for my grandfather—to actually get to such a level where he felt that suicide was his best and only option. To impress upon you how much it was swept under the rug just within our family, I only learned about his initial suicide attempt from my mother just a couple of years ago, in my late thirties (he died when I was eight). So for nearly thirty years, I had no idea he had attempted suicide. I later discovered some letters between the American Medical Association and my grandmother. In one letter my grandmother outlined some of the issues she felt contributed to his suicide—one of which was the substandard care physicians receive when confiding in physician friends while seeking medical care. The psychiatrist he sought out who told him to "suck it up" was a former colleague and friend. My next step, call it a goal, is to interview his last nurse, the one person who was perhaps closest to him when he committed suicide. I desperately want to understand his actions.

Ashley

* * *

December 5, 2015

Ashley,

Did you ever interview his last nurse?

Pamela

* * *

December 6, 2015

Dear Pamela,

Yes. I did interview his last nurse, and his last lab technician, and my mother, and my uncles, and some of his closest friends. I did so in order to better understand my grandfather's death. Being from a small town, so many rumors circulated around his death. The more disturbing one was that he could never have committed suicide and was murdered, perhaps by a disgruntled patient or as a result of a gambling debt. He was an avid gambler, among other things. But according to my uncle Bob (the oldest child of my grandparents' children) my grandfather had no gambling debts as his gambling was more of a recreational outlet.

When my grandmother awoke the morning after my grandfather had committed suicide in his car, she was immediately concerned because she could tell he had not come to bed that night. She looked out the front window and down to his car. She knew something had happened and immediately called his nurse. She found his lifeless body in the backseat of his car, told my grandmother, and then called the authorities who came down to do their investigation.

Because of the manner of his death, I knew an autopsy was done and, as morbid as it sounds, I tracked down a copy (not the pictures mind you, just the report). He had five gunshot wounds from an automatic pistol to his head and upper torso. What I found interesting was that none entered his cranium. The initial shot that took his life severed a vertebral artery. The other shots lodged in various places in his back and scapula. He had an entry wound by his ear. He also had evidence of diazepam in his system, the drug he had initially tried to overdose on in his first attempt. With the type of automatic weapon he used, the coroner, police chief, and investigator all agreed the manner was suicide.

When I mentioned that the circumstances surrounding his death were "swept under the rug," I did not mean that as a slight to my family. According to my mother's account of his initial attempt, it was downplayed by my grandmother, likely to protect their children from the harsh truth. My grandfather told his nurse and lab tech that he took too much Benadryl one night to help him sleep, and they believed him. As an aside, they both believe he was murdered, but his nurse's husband believes he committed suicide (he was one of my grandfather's close friends). So, you see, we often believe stories that are sometimes woven with threads of questionable truths. But to bring my point home further, I did not know of his first attempt until I was thirty-five years old and had returned home to start my practice. My mother told me the story on our way to visit an old family cemetery. I was floored. How could this have stayed "secret" so long? Why am I just now learning this? Again, I think it was because of the circumstances and how we as a culture deal with suicide.

Both the police chief who investigated the scene (who happened to be the father of one of my best friends and one of the most honorable men I've known) and the medical examiner himself deemed my grandfather's death a suicide. After having finally collected an overwhelming amount of details surrounding his death, from multiple sources, and even taking on the tedious task of procuring his death certificate, I now firmly believe he committed suicide. For what reasons, I do not know. Only my grandfather knows.

It is my belief he was profoundly depressed and did not get the help he truly needed. But you and I know that sometimes, despite the best treatment, you cannot stop a determined person who has the means to do so. Just prior to his first attempt, he had retired, then come out of retirement to practice again. Perhaps he did not know how to leave the practice of medicine and/or his patients who loved him dearly, maybe too dearly. Perhaps he saw some disease process in himself that he did not want to endure, but I find this hard to believe, because aside from the obvious traumatic wounds from the gunshots found at autopsy, he was the picture of health (he was an avid runner, golfer, tennis player, fisherman, and hunter). He had a tumultuous childhood with an overbearing father, but he also had the sweetest, most loving mother who likely helped him overcome the insecurities that his father dealt him.

In my humble opinion, the thing that doctors so deeply want to possess is control. Control over disease. Control over how a patient responds to a treatment. Control over how the patients flow into and out of your office. Control over what the patient knows about his or her illness. Control over how one dies—particularly how we, ourselves, die. Maybe his suicide was him exhibiting his last measure of control.

Ashley

* * *

December 6, 2015

Ashley,

I'm impressed by your investigation and your tenacity. Incredible how the truth can be hidden for generations.

As an aside, the more accurate terminology is "died by suicide" vs. "committed suicide." "Commit" implies that it is some sort of crime. It also reinforces the mental health stigma that keeps mental health questions on physician licensing and credentialing applications in the criminality section (along with questions about felonies and DUIs). The medical community and even news reporters continue to use stigmatizing terminology like "committed suicide" because suicide is still taboo, so we don't even know how to talk about it.

Thanks for being a truth seeker.

Pamela

17

Dee

August 18, 2013

Dear Pamela,

I didn't realize that so many others in the field suffered as I do. I have tried to get help many times but it's hard because I don't think that anyone takes me seriously and I don't think I can be completely honest with anyone without major repercussions. I don't have any friends to socialize with and all my relationships have failed. I come from a background where I was the first to get a higher education, so they think that I should be elated to just have MD behind my name and tell me to "suck it up." I don't want to possibly lose my license because honestly I love taking care of patients and sometimes that is the only time I get a few moments of happiness. But things have been so bad for me that I have resorted to just doing locums [fill-in work] so I can isolate myself because sometimes I can't stop the tears. I have tried [suicide] a few times and the last time probably would have worked; but at the time I was lying there looking at the dog I had then, who was curled beside me nudging me to get up. Somehow I drove to the ER, although severely hypotensive, where I was hospitalized and they chalked it up to the fact that I had not really been eating or drinking for weeks. I no longer have that fur companion so I find myself alone and thinking about an escape a lot.

Dee

* * *

February 26, 2014

Dear Dee,

I want to thank you for your story that you posted on my blog last year. I'd like to share your experience to raise awareness on the topic of physician suicide. The "suck it up" strategy isn't working, as you know.

Pamela

* * *

February 26, 2014

Pamela,

I had stopped believing in divine intervention, but maybe your email is some form of it or maybe it was a coincidence or maybe I am just crazy. When I commented on the blog, I used this email that I rarely check. I actually felt like I had just reached out to my family for the last time this morning because I had been through so many things in the past year and for some reason, checked this email and saw this message. Thank you for all of the work that you do. I very rarely reach out to anyone anymore but if it is okay I will ask one question. What do you suggest physicians that are in that dark place consistently do? Especially if they have a weak or nonexistent support group? The mental health system here is terrible. Most of the resources and funding has been cut. Most times I just don't know what to do any longer and don't know how to keep going. Sorry for the venting and I apologize if this catches you at a bad time.

Sincerely,
Dee

* * *

November 30, 2014

Dee,

I am checking in again. I have some more comprehensive answers to your question on how we can support each other in a lecture I just gave in DC for the American Academy of Family Physicians. "Physician Suicide 101: Secrets, Lies & Solutions" [see Resources] is now fully transcribed on my blog. Here are a few actionable steps from my presentation:

1) **Talk about physician suicide.** We must bring this conversation into the light of day. If we see a colleague who is struggling or having a rough day, reach out. If you are struggling, please ask for help.

2) **Stop the bullying and abuse.** We can all reach out to faculty who use shame-and-blame teaching. Call attention to the violence and offer alternatives. Fear-based teaching methods should never be used to "train" doctors.

3) **Learn nonviolent communication.** Why speak violently to one another? Nonviolent communication can reduce the trauma of our already traumatic jobs.

Pamela

P.S. I still highly recommend that you see a counselor and get a weekly massage. Don't isolate!

P.P.S. I think you need pet therapy. Go to the humane society and get a fluffy companion. :)

18

Amelia

December 6, 2015

Pamela,

I just wanted to touch base and let you know that I'm just finishing my last week of Ob/gyn and it was horrible! It was the first time in my clinicals that I was belittled and ridiculed and made to feel small and insignificant and just plain stupid. It was awful, I tried to stay strong, but I would leave the hospital after a delivery or C-section and just sob in my truck. A few times, after a late-night delivery I would cry myself to sleep. I will never be that type of doctor. My supervising physician sees about fifty to seventy-five patients per day in his clinic while also doing deliveries. It is an insane schedule and I've been on call 24/7 for the entire rotation! Which is totally against my school's policies, but my school doesn't ask for feedback and there is no way I am going to say anything—we're told to just "suck it up."

I have to say—dreaming about how different my clinic is going to be is what brought me through those dark days. I always try to take my time with patients and talk to them about everything that is bothering them and I hug them! You are my inspiration, and your life, your passions, your emails and Facebook posts are so important—don't stop doing what you're doing!

Amelia

* * *

December 6, 2015

Amelia,

Have you ever been suicidal or had suicidal daydreams through any of this mistreatment?

Pamela

* * *

December 6, 2015

For sure, Pamela!

Last week I was getting out of my truck and had the thought that I could so easily step in front of the car that was going too fast down the street. Everyone would think it was an accident. Then there are the thoughts of whether this was at all worth it—going back to school, leaving my job, my house, my support network, that just adds to the sadness. I've struggled with depression and although I have developed some really good coping strategies, this rotation has robbed me of a lot of joy. Thankfully, I am going home for three weeks and I'll be soaking up all the joy and happiness that I can from friends and family and especially all my little nieces and nephews!

Amelia

V

Occupational Hazards

We enter medicine with our mental health
on par with or better than our peers.
Suicide is an occupational hazard of our profession.

19

Ben

May 22, 2014

Dear Pamela,

I went through a malpractice trial. Worst experience of my life. I wanted to die. I was not trying to hurt the patient; I was trying to help. Major league baseball players get millions, and yet strike out, or have a ball bounce over their head. But physicians have to be perfect, all the time. And babysit. And entertain. What bothers me most is in the last ten years I was swindled by a real estate broker for a half a million dollars, embezzled by an employee, and they got treated better than I did in the malpractice system. Yet I was not trying to hurt anyone, or being dishonest, or stealing. When I am treated worse than a thief, or embezzler, it is frustrating. Frustration leads to depression, depression leads to hopelessness, hopelessness leads to suicide.

Ben

* * *

May 23, 2014

Ben,

We lose so many docs to hopelessness. We're held to an impossible standard. Patients want a human connection, yet we are not allowed to be human. Humans are imperfect and make honest mistakes.

Pamela

20

Philip

June 11, 2013

Dear Pamela,

I am still in a state of shock hearing that my brilliant, loving, compassionate, successful, well-respected, honest, hard-working physician committed suicide this past week. Pressure from the changing medical community and insurance [system] had forced him to close his thirty-year practice and he went home and shot himself in the head. The letters keep coming in of how many people loved him, were healed by him, and admired him. What a tragic end to a successful career. Everyone is asking why. He was the best of the best, surgeon and specialist, nice home, nice family and now he is gone. Totally tragic.

Diana

* * *

June 11, 2013

Dear Diana,

I know of your wonderful doctor, Philip Henderson, M.D., III, a fourth-generation physician, an obstetrician just a few hours down the road from me. I think he delivered more than 6,000 babies (that's like one-sixth of the town!). Typical of nearly all physician suicides, nobody sees it coming. Shocked, everyone is left to ask, "Why?" What a huge loss of a great physician who brought so many into this world.

Blessings to you,
Pamela

* * *

April 4, 2014

Pamela,

Reading all of these comments on your blog today took my thoughts back to a year ago when I found out my doctor had just committed suicide. Recently I made an appointment with one of his associates for my yearly exam and am hoping that perhaps she will be able to shed some light and help me understand. Yes, even a year later I am still saddened by the shortsighted actions that led to his death. My only conclusion is that perhaps he truly loved his exceptionally well-run clinic, reputation, patients, and work so much that at age sixty-five the concept of trying to "sell" himself after his clinic was forced to close was totally inconceivable. I wish he could have realized that his gift and skills could have worked absolute miracles in millions of places on this earth. We have been living abroad for two years. The field is open and there is so much need. There are so many other options where he could have found total joy and happiness doing what he loved to do.

I am grateful that you are being bold enough to raise awareness about this issue. I think that everyone needs a confidential shrink once in a while. Especially those who are in high-profile pressure positions—especially the medical community where people have to wear the badge of "super human" every day. How sad that we have created a stigma in our country labeling those who seek counseling or professional help as flawed, unbalanced, or incompetent. I believe those who are willing to look at their issues and work them through are the more intelligent sector who create a better life for themselves. Everyone needs someone from time to time who will hear their frustrations and their heart. Everyone needs someone to help them see where and how to improve the quality of life and living. No one should have to walk the path of life alone—especially because of their occupation or fear of being censured. No human being should feel so alone, pressured, and despondent that the only option is suicide. This is especially true for brilliant doctors who, generally motivated by a desire to serve and help other human beings, have sacrificed so much of their lives becoming experts in their field.

May you be blessed for bringing this issue to light and providing this forum for expression.

Diana

21

Hal

April 27, 2014

Dear Pamela,

I considered suicide for a period of several months in the fourth year of med school, seeing it as an exit option from an (nearly) intolerable present and daunting future. The scary thing (for me) was that it was not emotional; it was an analytical exercise.

Now, more than thirty years later, I find myself musing (not seriously yet) on suicide, and I'm in survival mode hoping to find a winning lottery ticket so I can retire. I think it is time for me to repeat previous therapy.

A decade ago, my distress was greater, as the sense of being trapped and harassed were worse. Relief came with a mission trip to do medicine in an impoverished country where I was rebooted. My dissatisfaction withered and my joy in medicine was restored, although the wearing down restarted immediately with my return. I intend to do more mission work overseas when I "retire," a better exit plan than I had in medical school.

Hal

* * *

April 27, 2014

Hey Hal,

So many docs feel trapped (student loans, assembly-line medicine, bureaucratic BS). The key is to have autonomy, be appreciated by patients, and do the work you love. Have you thought of opening your own clinic? It's easy! Mission trips are great, but you really don't have to escape the USA to live your dream in medicine. :)

Pamela

22

Hannah

October 6, 2013

Dear Pamela,

Having spent too many nights trying to keep my patients alive and well (being the doctor who delivered probably the most drug addicts in 2009) I found myself undermined by a religious health care system. I spent many nights hoping I would not be alive when morning came. This wasn't the life I wanted, but now I will suffer a few more years to provide for my family. My bankruptcy case is tomorrow and I hope at least I won't have to become a bum. How many doctors do I know who have committed suicide: seven. How many do I know who have contemplated suicide: four.

Hannah

* * *

October 6, 2013

Hannah,

I'm here for ya. Heading to the mountains today to lead another physician retreat. If you ever get a chance, you're welcome to join us. Love to meet ya.

Pamela

* * *

October 6, 2013

Pamela,

Wow! I thank you for being available. Back in my worse days there was nothing on the web. I appreciate your blog. At least I know I'm not alone.

Hannah

* * *

June 4, 2014

Hannah,

You mentioned knowing seven docs who died by suicide. Are you aware of their methods, genders, specialties? Any other docs you know who died by suicide? Please share what you feel comfortable sharing. I'm trying to track all these suicides. Nobody else seems to be tracking these suicides and we must know more about what is really going on and why.

Love,
Pamela

* * *

June 8, 2014

Dear Pamela,

Doc #1 Male, late thirties, crashed plane Gulf of Mexico (pediatric intensivist)
Doc #2 Male, fifties, gunshot to head (family doc), he also killed his family
Doc #3 Female, late fifties, ran car off bridge (Ob/gyn)
Doc #4 Male, fifties, gunshot to head (Ob/gyn)
Doc #5 Male, fifties, overdose (internal medicine)
Doc #6 Female medical student, twenties, jumper
Doc #7 Male medical student, twenties, gunshot to head

Although #6 and #7 were not "doctors," for all intents and purposes the stress of medicine killed them. In 1999 I heard four med students in Boston committed suicide, but nobody is counting how many medical students are committing suicide either.

Hannah

* * *

September 4, 2014

Hannah,

It's crazy! Nobody is tracking this data. A doc just told me that two third-year female family medicine residents in one program died in a suicide pact! Together. By overdose. And they also had a gun! Plus another doc killed himself in that residency. Ya think this residency program has been investigated? Unlikely. They just keep hiding the bodies. With an average of eight residents per class, they lost 25% of their students to suicide!

More than 400 US doctors die by suicide each year according to Medscape (that's like losing an entire medical school). Widespread under-reporting and miscoding of death certificates as "accidental" means the numbers are even higher. I've also heard reports that we lose 150 medical students per year to suicide. Given that a typical primary care doc has 2,300 patients under their care, that means more than one million Americans lose their docs to suicide each year! This is a huge public health crisis.

Yet nobody is compiling accurate data. It's not like we're migrant farmworkers. Everyone tracks our every move, our every prescription, every board score—until we die by suicide. Then it's like we never existed!

Just spoke to med students about suicide prevention. "How to graduate medical school without killing yourself" is filmed and fully transcribed on my blog [see Resources]. If you know premeds or med students, could you pass this along? Do you have any connections to med schools or residencies? I need to reach more students to stop this senseless loss of life—sooner the better.

Pamela

* * *

September 5, 2014

Pamela,

I do not know any med students. I am truly grateful for your mission. You helped me through some of my darkest hours just by being there. Maybe we can start a "save the doctors" movement.

Hannah

* * *

December 15, 2014

Dear Pamela,

I turned down a job today because it had a $500,000 life insurance policy. I knew I would become stressed and depressed and would have an untimely death so my daughter could finish college and I could end the pain. People who commit suicide don't do it to end their lives; they do it to stop the pain.

Hannah

VI

I Lost My Self

Our clinics and hospitals are filled with doctors who are
missing in action.

23

Beth

May 22, 2014

Pam!

No one looks at doctors as human. Must be that "salary" (the public needs more education about physician debt). Our time, our compassion are looked at as someone else's right! Now we may not even be able to be paid for our time but only for "outcomes" which we have little control over.

I lost my spouse to alcoholism. I was an abused teen. I am a great primary care doctor. But I am emotionally drained. Dangerously so. When my few but intense relationships fail, I feel like I have lost the tiny little bit of love and support "for me," and I contemplate suicide often. I resent patients. I resent my children. For sucking the emotional life out of me.

I feel doomed to always be the caretaker. But never be on the receiving end. To never have time to read a book, to truly relax, to have someone smile and spoil me! I'm not sure I could accept it. We are trained to be the givers. Not the takers. I'll always be essentially alone at the end of the workday. Until I die and that will be that.

My soul feels like it is shriveling up and dying, yet I show up to work and smile, love my patients, hold their hands when they cry, try to help them see that they are "okay." Everyone thinks I am an awesome doctor. I am. But I'm dying inside. I see it like an hourglass—blood dripping out, none going back in.

But no one sees me. I am one of those perfect doctor machines. I fail to exist except for what I can do for others. That is why doctors die. They care themselves into emptiness. And can't find their way back . . .

Beth

* * *

May 22, 2014

Dear Beth,

I recognize a version of myself in your letter. I think EMTs, nurses, veterinarians, dentists and others in the caring professions may care themselves into oblivion too. We carry the suffering of the world. That's what we are trained to do—without complaint. It can destroy us. You can heal. Can you work fewer hours? Go to a spa? Get a massage? Get a puppy? Call me! As usual, I'm overflowing with ideas . . .

Pamela

24

Teresa

September 26, 2015

Hi Pamela!

When my ex-husband was in medical school, his lab partner and friend (good buddy and mentor type) drove out into a field one day and shot himself in the head. We found out about it on Halloween Eve. My husband started to laugh; the strangest hiccupping sound I ever heard come out of his mouth. He never laughed any other way after that; he seldom ever laughed after that. He too struggled with depression and suicidal thoughts, as well as alcoholism and sexual addiction/multiple affairs. We were married twenty-one years and then he divorced me for someone ten years younger. He is estranged from his daughters, weighs close to 400 pounds, and I seldom see him. When I do, I get an overwhelming feeling of sadness for the slow suicide that is his life, for the beautiful man who is missing in action forever. He was a musician, a poet, a gifted singer, writer, and gardener—none of which he does anymore.

I hate medicine. It cost him his true life; it cost me and his daughters our family; it is the source of unending grief for me when I let it be; but I have worked hard to heal and have found ways to deal with my own mental health issues, ways to stay in recovery.

My daughters are adults now and are doing well, although some aspects of life are still a struggle. We can communicate about feelings, dreams, hopes, fears, and they have a step-dad now who they love immensely, who loves them unconditionally. And he's not a doctor.

I went on to earn a PhD in human studies and I research resiliency. I work in a mental health role. I write . . .

. . . and some days I still weep for the incredible losses the terrible Mistress of Medicine inflicts, and for the beautiful dream that disappeared.

Thank you for "listening."

Teresa

P.S. You may share my story if you think it will help someone.

25

Judy

November 18, 2014

Dear Pamela,

I was a near loss a few times over for my "chosen" profession. I went to medical school at the prodding of my family. I hated it and had a bout of depression while in the "booking stage" of school that I weathered without treatment. Somehow I kept passing my classes. I developed test anxiety along the way, which only made it worse.

With patients I found I had some natural ability and hand skills. I set a goal to graduate because no one gets credit in life for part of med school. I dealt with chauvinism and teaching by intimidation/shaming. That was how things were done at that time. Graduation felt like a sham. It did not mark pride so much as survival.

I had mild runs of depression on and off in residency, but was still functional and respected. To boot, I did it as a single parent of twins (my med school marriage didn't make it).

In private practice and dealing with the long hours and family strains, I continued to suffer mild burnout in waves. I continued. A few lawsuits (dropped) further stressed my system. Another lawsuit for a patient I saved ended in a settlement with my attorney saying they should have had a parade for me instead. More chipping away.

I allowed myself to become a salaried physician, and then had all my ability to control my career taken away. I was thrown into hospital and call-group politics. I grew to hate my job more and more. I became anxious about complications and things that could happen on my watch, even though I had a good track record. I dreaded call nights. I was crying in the call room wanting to go home.

Finally, I asked for leave, though I asked for family reasons, not my mental health, for fear of losing my hospital privileges. While I was on leave, the chair threatened to shut down my practice and did nothing to cover my patients. I sank into a suicidal place.

I went to Borders Bookstore to find the book *Final Exit,* to know how many of what pills it would take to kill myself. They didn't teach that in my training. Borders didn't have the book, so I stood with tears running down my cheeks in front of the Death and Dying section. A woman approached me and asked if I had lost anyone dear to me. Not being able to admit the truth to her, I said "yes," and let her hold me while I cried on her shoulder. Only later did I see the irony that I had lost me. I did find the book at the public library, but never went beyond that.

Judy

26

Sue

May 9, 2014

Dear Pamela,

I never thought I would have to be in this world alone, but as a physician I've found that any partner I had would leave, complaining that I worked too hard and did not bring home enough money. They would use my time at work to pursue other relationships, and I was expected to cook and clean when I finally got home. Some were physically abusive.

I came back East, and started a home birth practice that was my joy. Then the medical board went after me for supporting midwives. I was "on probation" for four years, and finally won, but at what cost? All physician jobs ask about board actions and mental health treatment.

I returned to my hometown and now have a small barter clinic. I make less than the poverty line, am now a single parent, and my son is on Medicaid and free school lunches. I have many patients who love me, and I recognize the relationship that you describe—house calls, laughing together, and true intimacy! When I go out in public, folks who hate doctors come up on the attack and complain about all of us rich, greedy doctors, how their lives were ruined by doctors, while they puff away on their cigarettes, swilling down their beer.

What then is the exit strategy? As the medical examiner, I see all the suicides. I don't want to end up like those poor torn-up bodies. I see the loving couples at church, and accept that there will be no Prince Charming for me. There will be no one to care for me when the breast cancer comes. There is no savings, no retirement. As I do house calls and care for the dying, I know that there will be no such loving doctor for me.

A married physician couple in the next town died of Botox overdose and three physicians' wives have died by overdose. Nice people don't talk about it, I am told.

Sue

* * *

May 9, 2014

Sue,

People have no concept who doctors really are—on the inside. Medicine is a labor of love. We give our hearts and souls and brains to our patients—often at our own expense. I'm here for you . . .

Pamela

VII

Existential Inquiries

Life is an enigma. So I went to medical school
to see if I could make sense of things.
Now I have more questions than answers.

27

James

April 5, 2014

Dear Pamela,

I suspect that you would be hard-pressed to find one of us who isn't at least sometimes suicidal. We're just not allowed to admit it as it would end our careers.

James

28

Kaitlyn

April 11, 2013

Dear Momma and Daddy,

I am so dreadfully sorry for the unimaginable pain and hurt that I have caused you by taking my life. I am sorry for hiding from you that I was so deeply sad. I am sorry for not letting you know that I felt like I simply no longer wanted to live my life. I am sorry that I did not let you in on my perpetual despair that I lived in. Depression is nothing new to me. I can't remember a time in my life in which I didn't feel like I was barely treading water. I never told you how pervasive it was because I wanted to protect you from it, and I wanted to protect myself from it. But I have finally decided that I'd rather just not exist. I have found myself happy on occasion, and I have had many pleasurable things in my life, but mostly I feel overwhelmingly sad and exhausted from the weight of it. I would just rather not endure it any longer. I would have died years ago, but I couldn't bring myself to cause you such sadness and heartache. I still can't bear to think of the hurt this brings you, but I just can't go on.

You both are the most wonderful parents on the face of the earth. Please do not blame yourselves. Please don't wonder what you could have done. The only thing wrong is me. I love you deeply. I respect you immensely. I wish I could have waited until you both had gone peacefully many years in the future, after you've fully lived your own beautiful lives, but forgive me that I couldn't. This is the worst thing I will ever do to you. I am sorry I cannot ever make amends. I just want you to know that I love you so very much and that even though I don't want to live, I still wish you all the happiness in the world, and I wish I could be able to have it with you.

I know you may not understand why I didn't seek help. I don't know if I can really explain why. I just want you to know that I may be incomprehensible and you may be angry with me, but I am not angry, and while it eludes me why I was destined to live the way I've lived and to feel the way I've felt, this choice makes sense to me. I know I had such a seemingly bright future, and I know I would have been such a successful doctor and wife and mother. But all I have ever desperately wished for is to not feel like not existing would be preferable to being who I am and living the life I live. But that's never been true. And that's deeply sad and horrible and possibly terribly unfair. But that is how I feel and how I've felt for longer than I can remember. It may be inadequate and it may not justify my action, but it is the best explanation I have.

I hope you will forgive me. I hope you can be happy again. I hope you can find the strength to endure this burden I've placed upon you. And I hope you will never doubt how much I love you.

Please take care of [my cat] Gatito. If you can't bear the thought of him living with you, please find him a good home. I know this will hurt him, but I want to limit that hurt as much as possible.

Please make sure the people to whom I have left letters are notified and that they receive my letters. Their phone numbers are listed below their addresses. You do not have to call them, but please make sure someone does.

I love you both so much.

Your Daughter,
Kaitlyn

* * *

May 31, 2014

Dear Pamela,

On April 11, 2013, I lost my twenty-three-year-old, brilliant daughter, Kaitlyn Elkins, to suicide. She was just beginning her third year of medical school at Wake Forest School of Medicine in Winston-Salem, NC. Saying we were and still are devastated is a great understatement, but another thing was the absolute shock as we thought she was one of the happiest people on this earth. She was sweet, brilliant, gifted in all academics as well as an artist, poet and writer, and marathon runner. And she never, ever in her whole life showed her depression to us (her parents) or her friends, except she did tell her last boyfriend that she was depressed at times, but she told him we knew. We didn't. I think she told him that so he would not tell us.

She was highly functional until the last day of her life, going to great lengths to plan her suicide and did it like a well-planned school project. She was doing very well in med school. She left us a two-page suicide note, as well as one to four of her friends and one to her sister. In it she told us she had been depressed all her life but hid it from us to protect us from it and to protect herself from it. She said she could not explain why she never sought help. She said she was exhausted from the weight of her depression and this is what made sense to her.

She always told us she loved medical school. I'm not sure, but since she said she had been depressed all her life, maybe medical school added so much stress that it made her depression worse. I think she never asked for help due to the stigma and she was a perfectionist and did not want to be seen as weak. She had to know, as well as I know, that depression is an illness, not a weakness and can be treated. But for whatever reason, she did not seek treatment.

She was an introvert, but did have close friends, but I don't think she had any in medical school. Whenever I asked if she had any friends in med school she said no, that mostly everyone went their own way. I did not worry about this, but in hindsight I think she felt lonely and isolated.

I had no idea that depression and suicide rates were so high in med students as well as MDs until she died.

I think as a child she must have suffered existential depression that so many gifted children suffer. Feeling alone because no one thinks as deeply as most people their age do, though I did not even know what existential depression was then, but only since her death I have researched this.

Med schools and the medical profession need to put more emphasis on mental health of their students and colleagues. They need to make it so no one fears losing their license by admitting they need help and getting it.

I just wanted to write to you because I am so glad you are bringing attention to this topic. I wish you continued success with this and maybe we won't lose as many brilliant med students and physicians that could have lived on and made a wonderful impact in our world.

Rhonda

* * *

May 31, 2014

Rhonda,

Oh, I would really love to speak with you. Thank you so much for writing me. I knew about your daughter, but I had no idea how to contact you.

Pamela

* * *

June 1, 2014

Hi Pamela,

Thank you for our talk last night. You are doing wonderful work and if I can help in any way, please let me know.

My grief drove me to writing and researching because I could *not* understand how someone so accomplished, who seemed so happy right up until the end, could kill themselves. I'm a nurse and I know the signs of depression very well. She never showed one single sign. I began on Facebook, then I started a blog to write about my grief. Soon I had an outpouring from some of her classmates and other doctors and residents. They told me how isolating medical school is. I also learned Kaitlyn probably did not seek help for her depression due to the stigma and fear that if she admitted to it, that it would ruin her medical career. I found out that any student or physician must report mental illness of any kind. That is why so many medical students and physicians take their own lives.

Kaitlyn was the brightest, most gifted person I have ever known and the joy of my life. Something must be done to end this stigma and to make it where doctors and students do not fear losing all they have worked so hard for. Thinking they will lose it all takes all their hope away, and what is life without hope?

I wrote a book about my daughter this past year. Another therapeutic way for me to get my feelings out, but it is also very much a warning to parents, teachers, counselors, medical students, and faculty that the very intelligent can be prone to existential depression and can hide their depression very well, a fact that very few people know. I will ship you a copy next week.

Rhonda

* * *

August 28, 2014

Rhonda,

[Posted to her Facebook page] I spoke about Kaitlyn [at my medical school presentation]. I will post video soon. I spoke about you as well and read your writing. And held up Kaitlyn's book. It was amazing. My first standing ovation! Nothing beats a room full of inspired medical students.

Pamela

* * *

September 1, 2014

Rhonda,

When you didn't "like" my Facebook post, your family knew something was wrong. You usually respond right away. I found out later that while I was inspiring medical students, you went missing. They found you the next morning. You died just like your daughter Kaitlyn, by suicide. I attended your funeral yesterday in Clarkton, North Carolina, where I met your kind family and dearest friends. I lost one of the sweetest people I never met. Rhonda, you touched me so deeply. Yet I could only touch your casket. Rest in peace, sweet, sweet soul. I'll continue where you left off with more devotion than ever. I'm here if you need me. XOXO.

Pamela

＊ ＊ ＊

October 28, 2014

Dr. Wible,

Thank you so much for your tireless crusade to educate educators, mothers, fathers, brothers, sisters, and all [people] about physician suicide prevention. Rhonda Sellers Elkins was my beautiful sister, whom I miss very much. She just could not go on in life with the guilt of not being able to see the lifelong depression that her daughter, Kaitlyn, suffered. Unfortunately, with Kaitlyn's depression, she chose the profession that was probably the worst she could have chosen. Everyone needs to know what goes on in med school and you, Dr. Wible, are truly making a difference. I say thank you.

Gail

VIII

Invisible Doctors

What does it mean when physicians are
unable to be seen as human beings?

29

Bruce

December 7, 2014

Pamela,

In anesthesiology, it seems we have a higher percentage of death by suicide than other medical specialties. My colleague took his own life over a year ago. I was basically okay until then, but it's how everyone reacted that really got me. The show must go on. We diverted patients the first night, probably because the ER had to see Joe when he came in. The next day all of us were back at work in the operating room. There was no time to grieve and we in the department were so stunned we did not know what we needed and what to ask for. It felt like abuse to not honor him or his colleagues with some rescheduling of operations. I will never be the same. I no longer see medicine as a force for good. It seems like it is a way for other people to make money off our talent, intelligence, education, or determination.

He was my friend!

Bruce

* * *

December 7, 2014

Dear Bruce,

I'd love to speak with you. As helpers we are not great at asking for help. Anesthesiologists are really high risk. Many reasons I'd like to share. Can you imagine if school shootings were handled the way doc suicides are? "Get back to class. Don't ask about Joe. Just do your algebra!" Let's talk soon.

Pamela

* * *

December 7, 2014

Pamela,

That would be excellent. Your article "Physician Suicide 101: Secrets, Lies & Solutions" [see Resources] was one of the first reports I have seen which really and bravely addressed this epidemic. I was relieved to see it in print. After Joe died last year, one partner fell ill, and two left the practice. Joe had been on call the night before the morning he hanged himself. He did it while his wife was at the grocery store with their youngest child. I'm okay, but really disillusioned about the world I worked so hard to join. I'm infuriated at the state of affairs in medicine, and wish I could open my own clinic, but I'm in the wrong field.

Bruce

30

Jennifer

December 16, 2014

Pamela,

Thank you for your writings and videos on physician suicide. I almost became one of your names in 2001 when I attempted twice to kill myself. These were not just gestures—they were well-planned but thwarted by several unexpected interventions.

Then several years later, a good friend, an orthopedic surgeon, killed himself by cutting his wrists with a scalpel. His name was Chad. I miss him to this day and wish I could have reached him but I know in my heart that when a person reaches that point, he/she is not reachable. The need to die is all-consuming and seems like the only relief possible from the deep, deep black hole that is beyond description.

I'm okay now after years of therapy and close psychiatric care. It also helped that I was finally diagnosed with bipolar type I and am now appropriately treated. It has made an immeasurable difference in my quality of life.

I don't think the public understands the severity of the pressures that a practicing physician faces. And I don't know how to make them—or, especially, my fellow physicians, understand. There is so much denial in the profession. I could go on and on about how I became the "invisible doctor" to my colleagues who would walk right by me without acknowledging my presence after my suicide attempts. I'd walk down the street, or go into a restaurant or movie theater, and there would be one of the doctors I used to work with. Before I could say anything, that doctor would turn aside or move away. It was bizarre. I had become invisible. Of all my colleagues, only two made contact with me to express their concern. One was Chad. Thanks for listening. If you ever want to contact me, feel free.

Jennifer

* * *

December 17, 2014

Dear Jennifer,

I'd love to talk to you. Curious if you could share more about the reactions among doctors to Chad's suicide and your attempts. I find the response from your colleagues both fascinating and extremely disturbing.

Have you heard of suicide censorship? It's when suicides are actively hidden from public view because they are considered harmful to others and politically incorrect by society, media, religion, hospitals, clinics, medical schools—even doctors.

When I began sharing my personal history as a suicidal physician, my brother told me not to talk about it publicly. When I've attended victims' memorials and medical society events for our many physicians lost to suicide, the word suicide is never stated aloud. Given the number of doctor suicides in town, I approached our newspaper to do a story. The reporter stated that their policy is not to report suicides unless the family wants it in the obituary. So I went to the TV station. They were mildly interested, but nobody wanted to talk. Even our medical society that spearheaded a wellness program for physicians would not speak publicly about physician suicide. The station wanted data. Catch-22. Data isn't being tracked. Nobody wants to speak. The stories died like the suicide victims—in secrecy and shame.

The fact is most physician suicides are not reported. When patients call for appointments, they're told, "Sorry, your doctor died suddenly." Hospital and clinic staff are instructed not to ask what happened to the suddenly missing doctor they knew and loved. Imagine if we handled Ebola or HIV with this level of secrecy.

Beyond censorship, I've been met with active criticism. When stating the manner of death, I've been accused of giving "gory details." Hit by a train, jumped from a hospital rooftop, overdosed in a clinic are not gory details. These are facts. Yes, method is relevant. And it varies by specialty. Yes, some specialties are higher risk than others. Yes, there is gender disparity. Male medical students and physicians die far more frequently than females. Yes, many choose to die inside clinics and hospitals. Yes, choosing suicide at work is significant. No, we will not be able to solve this if we do not talk about it.

Pamela

* * *

December 17, 2014

Pamela,

The reaction of fellow physicians was beyond belief. When my friend Chad committed suicide, the docs called for a big general meeting to help the physicians "deal" with this and talk about it. (No such response with my suicide attempts, other than a former call partner standing up and saying he wouldn't cover my call while I was out—even for the short term.)

At any rate, at this meeting about Chad, one of the things that several docs suggested was placing a memorial in the soon-to-be-completed break room for doctors. Everyone agreed this was a great idea, even to include a photo of him In Memoriam. A year or so later, I asked if this had ever been done, and I was told no, they decided they didn't want to be reminded of him. So much for physician denial—it's a tough nut to crack.

I'll look forward to talking with you. I'm way past my bedtime. What are you doing up at 12:20 a.m.? Aren't you a working woman?

Take care of yourself—if you don't, no one else will.

Jennifer

31

Paula

April 7, 2015

Pamela,

We've had three physician suicides in the thirteen years I've been at my job since leaving fellowship and I was shocked at how quickly they were given a cursory, sad nod, then forgotten. During medical school one classmate blew his brains out and it received barely a mention at the time from our professors. My husband, a health psychologist leading stress management workshops with medical professionals in our area, continues to report a great deal of frustration that "They won't talk and then it's too late!" Why?

As a physician in a high-stress job (who isn't, right!) covering two ICUs at a breakneck pace, I feel like I'm not allowed to fail, not allowed to have a bad day, and certainly not afforded an outlet if I somehow feel I am becoming compromised or just need some time off to rest (Heaven forbid!). There is no one to take our places.

Today my nurse practitioner called in sick and I realized—she can, but I can't. I absorb her work and press on. It's the unspoken law of the medical landscape and there's palpable resentment if another overworked doctor has to step in if you are somehow able to actually prove "Yes, I'm vomiting every five minutes and can't make it to the car." It can often feel like too much—especially when sleep deprived. There exists a breaking point and we all have one.

Recently I recognized the signs and it startled me—if one glass of wine calms the entangled fallout at the end of a day of difficult patients, families and unrealistic expectations around life expectancy, disease outcome, and cultural entitlement, then two does it better! Beginning to anticipate that "glass-of-friend" awaiting me at the end of a "document-this-right-or-get-prosecuted" day, I abruptly set it all aside for hot tea and orange juice. Honestly, it freaked me out how easily it happened that alcohol soothed and asked no questions—and how smoothly I justified it. If you don't think it can happen to you . . .

Paula

* * *

April 7, 2015

Paula,

Just read your letter which (of course) is spot on. I think physicians drink or use substances to dull the untreated mental anguish of our profession. Not like we can go get help without scrutiny. Physician licensing applications typically have that question about having ever sought mental health care. One doc in town checked the "yes" box because she got counseling during a divorce. Well the state mandated that she go to a psychiatrist to make sure she's not nuts before granting her a license. Geez! For marriage counseling! Non-punitive mental health care seems impossible for us to find, yet we've got easy access to liquor and firearms without scrutiny. In just over a year, we've had three physician suicides in my town. One bought the gun the same day, receipt still in the bag.

Pamela

32

Sylvia

December 9, 2015

Hi Pamela,

I am an anesthesiologist in the UK. I have struggled with my own mental health issues, including suicidal thoughts ten years ago. I have been greatly helped by the London-based practitioners health programme.

My hospital has once again had a trainee suicide last week, and of course there were "no signs" that he was struggling. Nice guy, worked Monday anesthetising gynae patients. Found dead at home Wednesday. Only in his early thirties. The work email used euphemisms like "sadly found suddenly dead at home." Who do these euphemisms protect?

Sylvia

IX

Physician Health Programs?

I assumed physician health programs
were health programs for physicians.
Now I'm not so sure.

33

Adam

March 24, 2015

Dear Pamela,

As a physician who struggles with suicidal thoughts, I appreciate what you do. Two years ago, I did a stint in a psych outpatient program due to depression, with great success. Since then I've moved to a new state and I find that I need support again. My medical director suggested I self-refer to the physician health program here. So I called (and didn't give my name) and was shocked by how unhelpful they were. They described the process, which would delay returning to work. I'd be forced to comply with years of monitoring and pay for multiple evaluations and random drug screens. (Even though I don't have a substance problem.) I may be mentally ill, but I'm not crazy! It seemed punitive and geared toward addicted docs with nothing to offer everybody else. I don't think preventing suicide is on their radar at all. I would love to do more to advocate on this issue, but honestly I'm just trying to stay alive.

Adam

* * *

March 25, 2015

Adam,

Other docs seeking emotional help for occupationally induced anxiety, depression, and suicidal thoughts have also been forced into Alcoholics-Anonymous-type, one-size-fits-all treatment programs (no matter their medical conditions). Some of these "health programs" are harming vulnerable physicians and should be investigated. Glad you didn't get caught up in the madness. I know of an excellent psychiatrist who drives 200 miles out of town, pays cash, and uses a fake name to get mental health care. It's sad when physicians feel they have to go underground with their psychiatrists to avoid professional persecution. I'm always here if you need to talk.

Pamela

34

Amy

October 11, 2014

Dear Pamela,

I'm amazed at the punitive terms I've had to face in recovering professionally from a depressive episode for which I was hospitalized last year. One of my requirements is to be urine tested for substance abuse, despite multiple demeaning assessments that have rendered the clear verdict that I don't have a substance use problem. I've had to attend costly treatments for "professionals" in which I am the only female in a group of male physicians who have had sex with their patients or have become assaultive with staff. Any efforts on my part to point out that I don't quite "fit" are taken as further evidence of my pathology. I'm a single parent as well, so that each of these "treatments" I'm required to attend takes me away from my two children for extended periods of time. Throughout all of this, nobody has told me how common my feelings are—that a large number of doctors feel depressed and suicidal at times. Rather, I've been told that my actions are unheard of for someone in mental health and may preclude me from ever providing therapy again since "we tell patients to never give up hope, but you did." Hopefully, in the near future this won't be a taboo subject, and there will be places for those like me to seek responsible and confidential care.

Sincerely,
Amy

35

Greg

June 22, 2012

Dear Some,

My family, I love you. To others who have been good friends, I love you too. This is just the end of the line for my particular train. Earth wasn't a great place for me. We'll see what else is out there. Will miss you all! I'm sorry, for what it's worth.

Love,
Greg

* * *

December 4, 2015

Dear Greg,

I feel like I've known you forever. This summer, I met up with Corinne, your friend who lived at the apartment complex where you died. She still feels guilty, like she could have stopped you somehow. I told her to let that go. Wasted energy. It's the physician health program that appears to have been the accomplice in your demise. How irresponsible that an organization would recommend that you not follow your psychiatrist's safety plan. Just hours later you were gone. Candles lit, music playing, surrounded by family photos, you slit your wrists and ankles in your bathtub. Must have been surreal to float away from the pain and leave your body. You were always a free spirit.

Meanwhile your mom has sent me your baby pictures, some of your elementary school homework, plus one of your crazy striped ties. She's still so devastated, though she finds comfort in sharing your life with me. She's even agreed to have your handwritten suicide letter on the cover of this book. Hope that's okay with you. :)

Met your sister Erica who carries around your ashes. I guess you know she's helping produce a film on physician suicide to honor you. So I have a sneaking suspicion that you're choreographing the whole show—especially after you spoke to my friend in a "dream." You told him, "I didn't kill myself. They killed me. I just finished the job."

Yep. Exactly. Just as I thought.

Pamela

P.S. Your mom first reached out to me in the letter below and then—after two interns jumped to their deaths from Manhattan hospitals within a few days of each other—your mom shared the following letter she submitted to the *New York Times*. Unpublished by them. Published by me. I got your back.

* * *

February 28, 2013

Dear Pamela,

Thanks so much for calling attention to this very real, and very serious issue. I am a physician (psychiatrist, fortunately) as is my husband. Our twenty-nine-year-old physician son died of suicide (now the more PC term that physicians should be aware of) in June of last year. We struggle every day to understand the "why" of this. As you point out in your articles, the causes and contributing factors are many.

He struggled with depression and alcoholism and was being monitored by the Missouri Physician Health Program. When he relapsed one week before he was to begin his oncology fellowship at a high-powered academic institution, he notified the board, then got drunk and took his own life (with a scalpel). No one at the hospital claimed to have any awareness of his struggles; worse yet, they cleansed the death notice we provided them of unsavory details. They clearly see his death as an injury to their institution. They have offered little in the way of condolence to us.

This matter must be brought into the light of day. The lack of data about the number of suicide deaths is appalling. The monitoring people from the medical board (who were the last to speak with him that day) have provided us with scant information. They told us that they did not plan any sort of internal case review. He was seeing a psychiatrist, but they never sought collaboration with him. They thought he was a "model patient." So this is what oversight by the medical board provides to impaired physicians. Well, I could go on and probably will but want to hear more from others. How can we take action? I cannot bear the thought of young doctors as dedicated and talented as my son dying in such a tragic manner. Your articles certainly resonate with Greg's struggle to come to grips with allowing himself to be human and vulnerable in such a highly competitive environment and to deal with the shame he felt about his very human vulnerabilities.

Karen

* * *

September 6, 2014

Dear Editor,

An unacknowledged predicament for physicians who identify their struggle with substance abuse and/or depression is that they are often placed under the supervision of their state medical board's physician health program (PHP).

My son, Greg, was being monitored by such a program. He took his own life at age twenty-nine, one week before he was to enter an esteemed oncology fellowship. His final phone calls were to the PHP notifying them of his use of alcohol while on vacation, a disclosure he had previously described as a "career killer."

These programs, which often offer no psychiatric oversight, serve as both treating and policing agencies, a serious conflict of interest. Threatened loss of licensure deters vulnerable physicians from seeking help, and may even trigger a suicidal crisis. Medical boards have the duty to safeguard the public, but the assumption that mental illness equals medical incompetence is an archaic notion. Medical boards must stop participating in the stigmatization of mental illness. We cannot afford to lose another physician to shame.

Karen Miday, M.D.

* * *

November 13, 2014

Greg,

Today is your birthday! They just happened to publish the article I wrote about you in Medscape today. Happy birthday, sweet soul.

You wouldn't believe how many of your friends and co-workers have written to me since I started writing about you! Everyone tells me how absolutely brilliant you are. Yeah, I knew that. The disturbing part is how our medical institutions dealt with your death. A nurse who adored you just wrote me:

> "I worked with Greg very closely. I knew he was not well and didn't say anything. That has haunted me, but mainly I wanted to state that when he died there was a lot of secrecy around the hospital as to how he had died and we (the staff) were instructed not to ask. I always suspected but never really knew what happened until I saw your article. While I'm still sad, I am relieved to stop wondering."

Incredibly disturbing how our medical institutions are so willing to cover up these suicides.

Hey, I keep sending your mom all your "fan mail." You have no earthly idea how many people love and miss you!

Pamela

36

Susan

November 21, 2014

Hi Pamela,

My ex-husband, also a physician, committed suicide one-and-a-half years ago. I have had my own episodes of depression with little support at work. (After taking three months off for a major depressive episode and to look after my grieving children, one of which was threatening suicide herself, I was told that I wasn't carrying my share of the load at work and had a "boutique practice." I'm a surgeon.)

It is a long overdue conversation that I am trying to start here in Canada as well. We, too, have a physician health program which is in conflict of interest as it pertains to licensing and physician support. To this point, they have focused mostly on physician substance abuse and disruptive behavior. These seem to me to be late stages of physician mental health problems. I would like them to deal with issues before they get to those stages. But it is hard to do until we "re-humanize" physicians. Any resources I can use to break down the silence and annihilate the taboo are appreciated.

Susan

* * *

November 21, 2014

Susan,

Totally agree that substance abuse and mental health struggles are late-stage consequences of decades of inadequate emotional support for the trauma we sustain in our daily work. There is power in numbers. We signed up to be healers, not victims. Let's start by protecting our most vulnerable physicians from persecution and mistreatment. Get active. Speak up. Do something. Anything.

Pamela

* * *

November 21, 2014

Thanks Pamela!

I've recruited three other physicians to help me. And we are meeting with our PHP. I'll keep in touch.

Susan

Part Two
Solutions

X

You Are Not Alone

If you made it into medical school you're already
in the top 1% of compassion, intelligence, and resilience.
You have no resilience deficiency. You're not defective.
You're responding normally to an abusive medical system.
So are your peers (who are also hiding their tears).

37

Norah

November 30, 2015

Dear Dr. Wible,

I saw the livestream of your TEDMED talk on physician suicide and I cried. To have someone acknowledge the desperation I feel was a luxury for the first time since almost everyone around me seems to be coping just fine and the only problem is me.

I'm in a developing country and thus you can add poverty to the misery of this career. I never knew saving 100 wouldn't make it worth losing one patient. I've been gradually losing the joy of life, the desire to talk to anyone, and the desire for life itself over the last few months owing to what I see every day: death, poverty, pain, turning away the dying because you have no room, inhuman coldness in dealing with patients, and on top of all that comes the life of a med student. I'm expected to stay up most of the week, blind myself with hours of studying (so I don't end up killing someone as we're constantly told), do nothing but study! I have no time for my family who live in the same place as me, no time for anything that defines me, no time for even lying in bed to think before I sleep. I'm simply operating on autopilot, trying to do what's expected of me and, when I can't, I have to grieve in silence.

I truly no longer know how to go on with my life.

Norah

* * *

November 30, 2015

Norah,

You are not alone. Do not give up hope! I'm sending you some inspiration. Check out "Our special message of hope for medical students & doctors" [see Resources]. Please know that we all support you and want to help you retain your humanity amid the suffering. You can reach out to us! Happy to FaceTime or Skype with you!

Pamela

38

Jessica

July 3, 2014

Dear Pamela,

I am a doctor who was nearly successful in "completing" my suicide ten years ago. After swallowing a carefully calculated lethal dose of a common analgesic, with extra "just to be sure," in combination with something to make me drowsy, I fell into a coma for twenty-four hours. I evidently then had a seizure and fell out of my bed. My then-fifteen-year-old son who was supposed to be staying with a friend stayed home from school and had picked open the lock to my room to see me. With the door open, he heard the fall and other noises that accompanied the seizure (I have no recollection of this). He dialed 911 immediately. I was very close to death. (He and my other child were in counseling after my attempt, as of course was I.)

If I could impart any wisdom, it would be this: Do not worry in the least what other people will think of you if you turn your back on a career or a lifestyle that is killing you. Take care of yourself and your children. Work half time and live in a small house or (gasp!) an apartment. Find another career or another version of doctoring. Don't get owned by your possessions, by the expectations of others or an image others conjure up when you tell them you're a doctor. The image is their burden, not ours, not mine. Trying to live up to the expectations of others almost cost me my life. That will never happen again. I now see the ways in which doctors are both admired and pressured by people who know nothing about us other than our titles—and try to steer clear of either.

After my attempt I searched and searched for any literature on near or "uncompleted" suicides. I found one little book with three examples in it in my local bookstore. That was it, and my search was not limited to physician suicides. I read that book over and over. I so understood those stories. Pamela, you will be doing an invaluable thing by collecting and assembling stories of near suicides. For someone like myself, who didn't think I was even depressed and thought I would never take my life, I had to know if there were others like me. There was something very comforting in knowing there were—even if it was only three.

Jessica

* * *

July 3, 2014

Dear Jessica,

The professional image of a doctor that we're forced to conform to is a prison. We are human. We are social animals. We need each other. I am assembling these suicide stories as you suggest. I've got far more than three examples of "uncompleted" suicides. Many more have daily suicidal daydreams. You are not alone, sister.

Pamela

P.S. I work part-time in my solo clinic and live in a small house. Best. Decision. Ever.

P.P.S. I work full-time on physician suicide. No pay. Labor of love.

39

Chris

December 3, 2015

Dear Dr. Wible,

I'm not sure you read your [Facebook] messages but feel compelled to thank you. I was finishing term two of med school and had a bottle of Xanax in my hand. I was ready, as so many of us are. I took three then three more and came across this link, "How to graduate medical school without killing yourself" [see Resources], which I believe may have saved my life and a couple of close friends who are also suffering. I'm near the top of my class and praying for death to escape the trap I'm locked into. I was in true delirium from lack of sleep and fear of failure. Studying in my sleep and waking up every hour in panic. Med school is doable but why must it be taught in this format? I read your stories and I'm just in shock how many others feel like I do or I feel like they do. Please keep sharing. You are saving lives, friend.

Chris

XI

Ask for Help

It's okay not to be okay.

40

Matthew

June 21, 2014

Dear Dr. Wible,

I am in great pain, suffering with suicidal thoughts. It's not imminent within the next seventy-two hours or so; I don't have access to lethal means in my apartment. But I wondered if you would be willing to listen. Even if it was just a brief email. I read your blog over and over. Like so many, I devoted my life to helping others, and I feel so profoundly punished. Thank you in advance.

Matthew

P.S. The irony is I am giving suicide prevention lectures while planning how I'm going to jump off a bridge. I was just sitting with a "suicidal" patient and his family thinking there's one of us who is suicidal at this table and it is not my patient.

* * *

June 22, 2014

Matthew,

Please give me your phone number and I will call you today. I'm happy you are asking for help!

Pamela

41

Zelda

November 12, 2014

Hi Pamela,

I read your article in the *Psychiatric Times* about doctors committing suicide. At one point you mentioned that a doctor saying, "I had a rough day" is code for *"I need help!"*

I'm not a doctor (dropped out of second year med school due to depression), but that very much applies to me. When I'm feeling at my worst it is somehow hardest to ask for help—maybe because I know not getting it will hurt more than I can handle, or maybe because I'm afraid that people actually will try and help. Whatever the reason, I think I need some advice on asking for help.

Usually when I try to ask people for help they don't seem to react, and I can't tell whether I'm not being clear enough or whether they just don't feel like dealing with a crisis. I often go into joking mode when I'm feeling at my lowest. Maybe that confuses people. I think the furthest I've gone in asking for help is saying things like "I really feel like I'm about to lose control" or "It's hurting more than I can deal with right now." But usually when I say something serious like that people seem to become less willing to spend time talking to me, and not more.

The other reason I'm highly unlikely ever to tell someone I really feel like killing myself is that it seems to be logically inconsistent. If I really wanted to kill myself, would I tell someone who would probably try to stop me? Catch-22 situation: if I'm rational enough to ask someone to stop me from killing myself, I am probably rational enough not to do so. It then starts to seem like my only reason to tell someone "I'm strongly tempted to kill myself right now" would be to get them to spend time talking to me about my feelings, which might come across as sort of needy and/or manipulative.

To sum up: I don't know how to ask for help with suicidal feelings. I don't know who it's okay to ask, when it's okay to ask, or how explicit I should be about it.

I'd really appreciate some advice.

Best regards,
Zelda

* * *

November 12, 2014

Dear Zelda,

How to ask for help in three simple steps:

1) Be really direct when you communicate. Be clear, precise, and honest. Simply ask for the specific thing that you need, such as "I need help coping with school" or "I need help with my relationship."

2) Ask the right person for help. Someone who does not look like they are in a hurry. If you ask other injured or suffering people (like suicidal physicians or med students with PTSD), it may be really hard to get the help you need. Best to ask those who are equipped with time, energy, and skills to help you.

3) Practice asking for help. Try it with someone today. Practice and you will get better at it. Since you are a "helper" by nature, this is not coming naturally—yet!

If you wish to know what people are thinking, just ask them, "What are you really thinking when I say this?" Does that help?

Pamela

* * *

November 12, 2014

Hello Pamela,

Thanks very much for the advice. But so then after saying "I need help," what do I say next that won't freak people out but will still lead to me getting some sort of help? Not freaking people out and getting help with bad feelings seem mutually exclusive to me at the moment.

Zelda

* * *

November 20, 2014

Zelda,

Tell them what you're thinking. How else will they know what you are thinking if you don't tell them?

Pamela

* * *

November 20, 2014

Pamela,

Okay, so I actually have to tell them something like "I'm thinking about killing myself?" That's really hard to say. I've tried telling people about my suicidal thoughts indirectly so many times. They mostly say things very similar to "You'll get over it."

But maybe I'm not asking for help properly. So what exactly am I supposed to say? I sometimes tell people "I feel really bad" and then they try to get rid of me as quickly as possible. Or they act like I'm doing something immoral by feeling bad. My psychiatrist usually reacts in a nice way, but often he's tired and doesn't look at his phone when he's not on call.

I'm going to try go to sleep now.

Zelda

* * *

November 28, 2014

Hi Pamela,

So I had an appointment with my psychiatrist this evening. He's not a very directive guy—very non-pushy when it comes to giving advice—and so this time I bugged him until he wrote down clear instructions for me regarding what to do in an emergency. I basically have to beg him to be bossy sometimes! So it turns out that, among other things, he suggested what you suggested: just say, "I need help."

Zelda

42

Mary

September 18, 2015

Pamela,

I just lost another colleague today. He is the second one in two months. He didn't show up to work and was found dead on his couch. It was obvious he was sickly for months, but he just kept going. I don't know if the autopsy will find suicide or cancer or something else. Either way if it was suicide by drugs or suicide by self-neglect, I'm tired of losing people and scared of being the next victim of this epidemic. What is there to do?!

Mary

* * *

September 18, 2015

Mary,

What do you think would help you?

Pamela

* * *

September 18, 2015

Pamela,

I don't know what would help. Taking care of the sick is hard enough without all the administration and profit-motive pressures from the outside world. I've seen people harden themselves, but lose empathy for the humans we care for. The only thing that I can think of to help myself is to pay off my loans, my mortgage, and create a decent college fund for my kid—then *get out* of the world of medicine.

Mary

43

Kelly

November 3, 2013

Pamela,

I am a Midwestern family physician who attempted suicide almost two years ago, shortly after starting a new, stressful position and then subsequently discovering my husband of eighteen years was having an online affair. I had been teetering on a fine line with depression and suicidal ideology for many years, and my resources had simply been used up. I carry more shame than I feel I can bear sometimes, and occasionally surviving seems like a curse. I have continued counseling and medication to fight the battle against depression, but I've had a hard time keeping my marriage together while doing a demanding job. Recently, I became somewhat overwhelmed at my work, and got teary. I told my boss I needed a minute (it was the anniversary of my attempt), and instead of letting me have the five minutes I needed to collect myself, he called in a colleague and told me I needed to go home. Granted, I work in a busy urgent care, but I didn't think it merited the threat of firing me.

Kelly

* * *

November 3, 2013

Kelly,

Regardless of his reaction, it was healthy for you to ask for help and ask specifically for some time for yourself. Caring for yourself and asking for what you need is a strength and not a weakness.

Pamela

P.S. Crying is nothing you need to hide. Crying is healthy. We should be very concerned about our colleagues who have lost their ability to cry.

XII

Survival Stories

Having survived, I now serve others.

44

Mark

May 22, 2014

Dear Pamela,

I entered recovery in 1996 in a five-month rehab program. I used alcohol, narcotics, and most anything else to change the way I felt. Returning to work resulted in three trips to psychiatric lock-down units. I spent a summer in bed. Didn't practice for a year. Was in my garage with a rope around my neck.

Therapy, support groups, medications, family love have helped control my diseases. I continue to see my psychiatrist quarterly and take my prescribed three antidepressants/mood stabilizers. Support meetings at least once weekly and retreat experiences quarterly. Actively pursue recovery and helping others.

Along the journey, I have bought my solo practice and just finished a two-year stint as Chief of Staff at our hospital. I take joy in attending support meetings in the same room where I chaired Med Exec meetings.

I share my experience, strength, and hope very selectively with colleagues, patients, and anyone else I think may benefit. I carry no shame but caution about public naiveté and professional ignorance.

I am forever grateful I removed that noose and got down off that ladder and have pursued life. It involves a lot of work, but I am rewarded daily.

Any way I can assist? The loss of an entire medical school on an annual basis is truly saddening. I am grateful to be one who got off the ladder. Are there many stories of survival?

Mark

45

Matt

April 14, 2015

Hi Dr. Wible!

First, let me thank you for your time and efforts in preventing physician suicide. I, too, recently was on the brink of suicide but fortunately, with the help of a long-time mentor and friend, I'm still here to write this letter. Currently I'm in my third year of my Hematology/Oncology fellowship at Brooke Army Medical Center in San Antonio.

My past has been filled with success but always hiding what I thought was a dark secret: depression. Previously my depression manifested as anxiety which I could channel towards hours of study which led to success. I'm not trying to boast but I was very successful: valedictorian in high school, finishing summa cum laude from Seattle Pacific University, and completing medical school second in my class (and class president). I went on to get my first choice of internal medicine residency in San Antonio and then was selected as the only Hem/Onc fellow for the Air Force in 2012. And all along the way driven by my anxiety and underlying depression.

Then fellowship started and things changed without me even realizing it. Anhedonia [inability to feel pleasure] set in. I got behind in clinical notes, stopped studying, couldn't retain information, and began to fail rotations. I couldn't understand what was wrong with me for nearly a year and a half. I was walking around in a fog. It was a vicious cycle that led me to the deepest, darkest point in my life. One night back in October after work, I sat in my desk for nearly an hour contemplating hanging myself in my office. The one thing that held me back was my three boys—it wasn't fair to them to grow up fatherless. But how did I get help? I finally was able to let my friend and mentor in my department know of my struggles and suicidal thoughts. I thought he might understand as he had just lost his physician brother to suicide. Long story short, I was allowed to leave the program and entered into a partial hospitalization program in town for six weeks. I also found amazing help and support with our psychologist. Without those two (and my kids) I may not be here.

It's been a long road (and will continue to be) but things are improving. Back in November I read your article "Physician Suicide 101: Secrets, Lies & Solutions" in Medscape which hit me hard. I have a new outlook on life and want to take this pile of manure and produce some fruit! I want to help break the stigma of physician depression and help those who may be where I was. Our department has recently asked me to share my story with incoming interns/residents in June (we had an intern suicide this past year). If you have any thoughts on how best to use my ten minutes, I would appreciate it. I want to join you in preventing what nearly cost me my life. Sorry for the long letter but I hope I hear from you soon.

Thanks again,
Matt

* * *

April 14, 2015

Matt,

Here's what to do in your ten minutes: share your heartfelt story. Be vulnerable. Medicine is an apprenticeship profession. We learn how to be doctors by studying doctors. Your story will help others open up and share their feelings. If possible, offer a panel discussion for residents during orientation. Allow other respected and successful physicians in your institution to share their experiences with despair openly so as to normalize our very human experience of anxiety, depression, and suicidal thoughts.

Pamela

* * *

April 14, 2015

Pamela,

Thank you so much for getting back to me so quickly and for the voicemail. I agree with you 100%. We have to stand up and express what we are going through to normalize our thoughts. You're right, we are not alone. That's exactly how I felt: alone with no options to get out of what I was feeling. I was afraid of the stigma, afraid of stepping away (and the program extension that would follow), afraid of feeling weak, afraid of being neglected by my peers. What has been amazing is the support I have received from my peers when I have told them my story. They truly were empathetic and many times had close family or friends who tried suicide or completed it.

I want to put a face and name to depression/suicide. I've been here six years and never heard another intern, resident, or staff speak of their struggles. As military we are required to undergo standard (and very ineffective) suicide awareness training. I want more than that. I want to verbalize it for others to "normalize" the feelings as you say; and I'm willing to be that person. I'm tired of trying to hide it. If I can help one other person step forward for help, then my mission will be successful. I'm pretty sure Alex has reached out to you as well. He is my mentor and friend I spoke of earlier who lost his brother to suicide around the time I was in despair (his brother had just graduated radiology residency). Together, I'm confident we can help by creating a family atmosphere in our institution. I also love your idea of starting a panel. I welcome any and all recommendations. If I can ever help you out in any way, let me know. I've found a new purpose for the future while going through my recovery.

Again, thanks.
Matt

46

Laura

December 22, 2014

Dear Pamela,

I am a family physician in the UK. I've been working as a full-time partner in a practice since 2006. I'm done in. I wanted to save the world. As a little girl, all I ever wanted to be was a family physician. At med school, I was annihilated by those clever doctors but carried on. Slowly but surely, seeing one patient every five or ten minutes for every hour of my working life, hitting government targets for just about every disease area, and having no time for myself (I've got two daughters eight and two years old) or my husband—I was utterly burned out. One of my partners, Peter, went off with stress, and on the day his sick pay ran out, was found dead in his closet by his teenage daughter. One of my brightest contemporaries, a witty, curly-haired redhead called Morgan, jumped off the cliffs into the sea.

Two years ago I was planning my own demise. I've never been to New Orleans but my plan was to drive to Manchester, get on a flight, book myself into the Lookout Inn, then get a gun and shoot myself in the head. I wanted to be far away from my family so that they couldn't stop me.

But I told my husband. I also emailed the Samaritans. I told my parents in a very roundabout way that I was having a very hard time. I'd seen how Peter's death had blasted a nuclear shock wave through a community.

But boy, did I feel like an utter failure. And now, one year later, as I'm about to leave my partnership after ten years, the other partners know that I couldn't hack it, couldn't take it, couldn't withstand the pressure. But they haven't helped, they haven't listened. I haven't had any time off!

You are a shining light of hope and I'm so grateful to you.

I try to be an excellent physician and really my only skill is listening. I try to do it well. My patients are often grateful but my partners aren't because they don't like listening, they don't like sharing themselves.

I don't usually like other doctors because they are so closed, so insular, and so unforgiving of weakness. But when I tell people that I can't hack it, that I'm leaving and going freelance, that I'm going to teach communication skills and do anything else that might help, they tell me I'm brave, that I am courageous, that they wish they could do the same.

But I'm not brave. I just didn't want to leave my two daughters without their mother the way that Peter left his four children without their father. I knew I just had to keep going. And that even if we end up living in a one-room apartment, we will still have each other and I will still be able to hug my kids and my husband. It was about survival.

I have talked to my patients and told them I am leaving because my job as a GP in the UK is impossible in its current format. There is no other option in the UK at present. People want the kind of ideal medical clinics you are designing in the US, but the NHS doesn't want that. It wants industrialized cheap one-size-fits-all medicine. It doesn't want activists and pioneers.

I am coaching doctors as part of my new freelance life—offering myself as a listening retreat, creating space for them. It is an amazing, transformational space and I just love it!

You just keep going, girl! And be so so proud of what you are doing.

Best wishes,
Laura

XIII

Community Action

Let's create a world where nobody has to write a suicide note.

47

Karyn

September 6, 2014

Dear Pamela,

You were there for me when I needed you, and likely saved me from becoming yet another statistic. I have a rare heart disease, and the unrealistic pressure of my job was literally killing me. I had stopped all of my medications for nearly two weeks literally hoping for the inevitable. Instead, I just endured an accelerating pattern of angina, anxiety, and migraines, which just fueled my desperation to put an end to it all.

I have restarted all of my medications and awaken each day grateful for the gift of life. In part, I owe that to you. For a time, my demons took charge and I was ready to concede defeat. Because you took the time to contact me on that pivotal day in my own tumultuous journey, I have the courage to go on. Day by day, one step at a time, I think I can. Thank you for being there for me and so many others in peril. Those of us who spend our lives on the edge, literally dying to heal.

Fondly,
Karyn

* * *

September 6, 2014

Karyn,

I am wondering what we can do as a community to save others in medicine. I think giving hope is often more important than any drug. What are your thoughts?

Pamela

* * *

September 6, 2014

Dear Pamela,

Suicide is rampant in our society itself, and none of us want to broach the topic. A frank discussion about suicide needs to be a mandatory part of the core curriculum in medical school. As a portion of that course, each student should meet with a guidance counselor or physician mentor, someone who will be available to them throughout their years of study.

We must remove the stigma of depression and mental illness and bring humanity back to the practice of medicine. As a profession, we must draw the line in the sand and say no to insurance and pharmaceutical companies. We can and must publicize the human tragedy of American medicine and offer a better collaborative alternative to the cookie-cutter approach. Every protest movement begins with a single voice of reason. It always seems an insurmountable challenge. But one voice added to one voice and so on becomes an unstoppable movement of change and liberation for us all.

Karyn

48

Kevin

May 24, 2015

Hi Pamela,

Thanks so much for contacting me! Our son Kevin passed away last month so we are still in a state of shock. The more I learn about this issue, the angrier I become that we felt so helpless to intervene and get him the help he needed. Missouri State Representative Dr. Keith Frederick contacted us the day after our son's memorial service and filled us in regarding House Bill 867 that would facilitate the screening of medical students for depression and other mental health issues. Knowing that you and Keith are out there trying to do something about this terrible problem gives us hope and strength that we can effect some change.

My husband, John, and I would be more than willing to do anything we can to help advance this cause. Below is a copy of my letter that Keith provided to the Missouri Senate since we could not be there to testify.

We would very much like to meet you when you are in St. Louis.

Many thanks,
Michele Dietl

* * *

May 7, 2015

Dear Senator Dempsey,

It is with a heavy heart that I write to you today asking you to please bring HB 867 to the Senate floor. As I sit writing this on a beautiful spring day, there is a hole in my heart that only a mother can feel while grieving for a lost child. Not just any child, but a promising young fourth-year medical student who was due to graduate on May 16th but who instead took his life less than two weeks ago after losing his battle with major depression.

As any one of the over 300 mourners at his service can attest, Kevin was an articulate, jovial, inquisitive, very special young man who truly went into medicine to help others. Looking back, it is apparent that he suffered from some depression throughout the long, lonely hours of medical school where he became isolated from friends and family while studying and making his way through the rigors of the medical school curriculum. It was not until a few months ago that major depression set in and would not let go.

I can never say for certain if this story would have ended differently had HB 867 been in place, but I believe Kevin would have been able to seek treatment sooner and our family would have had some resources in place to help us through this terrible ordeal. Kevin was petrified to seek treatment for fear it would have jeopardized his schooling and his future career in medicine. As parents, we were lost and didn't know where to turn. We were fearful to step in and notify the school of his troubles for fear it would keep him from the career he had worked so hard to achieve.

I beg you to please embrace this bill and raise awareness of this important issue so that other families will have the resources that were not there for us. We hope and pray that this bill goes through so that other families will not have to endure this unbearable pain.

Sincerely,
Michele Dietl

* * *

March 16, 2015

Dear Honored Members of the Missouri State Legislature,

I'm Dr. Pamela Wible, a family physician in Oregon. I've submitted my CV, witness form, and transcript of my testimony to Chairman Frederick. My schedule prevents me from traveling to Missouri for today's hearing; however, I thank Vice Chairman Morris and the Committee for allowing me to testify remotely in support of House Bill 867, legislation that would require Missouri medical schools to screen students for depression and offer mental health referrals for those at risk.

Medical students face enormous stress. Their workload and debt load are immense. They witness incredible human suffering with no emotional support or debriefing. Routinely sleep deprived, they're groomed in a medical culture that rewards self-neglect and often condones bullying.

Medical students are afraid to seek help for fear of retaliation or discrimination. Medical students are afraid to seek counseling because medical boards like the one in Missouri ask applicants if they've ever been treated for mental health issues. Checking the "yes" box can lead to a subpoena of one's "confidential" medical records.

Medical students enter medical school with their mental health on par with or better than their peers. Up to 30% develop depression and 10% become suicidal during each year of medical school. Both men I dated in medical school died by suicide. Depression and suicide are known occupational hazards in medicine.

More than 400 US doctors die by suicide annually. Widespread underreporting and miscoding of death certificates suggest the number is closer to 800. That's like losing all 391 medical students enrolled at the University of Missouri Columbia School of Medicine plus the 433 students at the University of Missouri Kansas City School of Medicine—every year!

Please join me in support of House Bill 867.

House Bill 867 benefits medical students. This bill will de-stigmatize mental illness and normalize medical students' rights to request and receive confidential mental health care. Student participation is voluntary and student data remains anonymous unless students select otherwise.

HB 867 benefits families by making mental health data transparent across all six Missouri medical schools. In medicine, informed consent is the standard of care, yet medical students and their families have not been informed of the health risks of a medical education.

Last fall, I attended a funeral. Kaitlyn Elkins was a star third-year medical student described by her family as "one of the happiest people on this Earth." She died by suicide, but the funeral wasn't for Kaitlyn. It was for Rhonda Elkins, Kaitlyn's mother. Unable to recuperate from her daughter's suicide, Rhonda took her own life. I asked Rhonda's husband, "If Kaitlyn worked at Walmart, would she and your wife still be alive?" He said, "Yes. Medical school has cost me half my family."

HB 867 also benefits patients. The best way to care for patients is to first care for our doctors-in-training. Let's practice what we teach. By truly caring for our medical students we demonstrate how we expect them to care for patients. The cost of not caring for our young doctors-in-training is more tragedy. Each year more than one million Americans lose their doctors to suicide.

Finally, I support House Bill 867 because it benefits medical schools. We teach medical students the value of evidence-based medicine, but if our medical schools are exempt from collecting evidence on medical student depression, how can we evaluate student mental health? How will we know the impact of medical school wellness programs? The psychological wellbeing of Missouri medical students is just as important as their academic performance. This bill finally gives us the data we need to properly care for and educate the future physicians of America.

On behalf of all medical students nationwide, I thank you for your support.

Pamela Wible, M.D.

* * *

June 16, 2015

Dear Michele [Kevin's mom] & Karen [Greg's mom from chapter 35],

This is an email I got today from a doc in her late fifties:

> "I saw that the last posting from you on physician suicide was [about] a young man from St. Louis. I know how terrifying it is to come to the end of medical school and know that you will have to be an intern. The fear is overwhelming at such awesome responsibility. I went to medical school here in St. Louis at one of the top ten medical schools in the country. And all of those smart people were terrified. At that time, there was no lottery in Missouri. They would take turns crossing the river into Illinois to buy lottery tickets hoping that if they won, they could wipe out their medical school debt and not have to be an intern."

We can create a more humane medical education system. I am devoted to accomplishing this in honor of your two amazing sons, Kevin and Greg [both died in St. Louis]. Sending you both LOVE!

Pamela

* * *

June 16, 2015

Oh my gosh ladies!

This is just so shocking to me and so incredibly sad. Pamela—thanks for forwarding. Words cannot express how thankful I am to you for working so hard to change the system in memory of our beloved sons.

Love to you both,
Michele

* * *

September 6, 2015

Hi Pamela,

We went up to get Kevin's diploma and met with both of the deans. It was, of course, a bittersweet day—so proud of the beautiful diploma he earned yet so extremely sad. They were very cordial, not surprising. I told them that I had been in contact with you and have learned so much about physician mental health issues in the last few months—things that I wish I had known sooner. I told them how appalled I am at the state of affairs in medicine and they acknowledged that it is a most difficult time to be in health care. I asked them what they are planning to do differently this year to help avoid another tragedy. They mentioned a few things such as doing away with class rankings—although I feel like House Bill 867 is what will catalyze widespread change. Hope all is well with you

Hugs,
Michele

* * *

December 27, 2015

Hello Pam,

As you know we had unanimous approval by a joint committee of the House and Senate to a compromised version of HB 867. Medical school lobbyists chose not to testify against HB 867 in public hearings, but instead used their considerable influence in the Capitol to prevent its passage. In a letter opposing HB 867, jointly authored by all six Missouri med school deans, they asserted that "Reporting the depression rates at our institutions will not reduce students' risk of depression, and we fear it actually perpetuates the stigmas associated with diseases of mental health." Why would they claim this? In my opinion, they are scared to death that the prevalence of depression among their students will be shocking and embarrassing to their institutions.

Medical schools should be assessed not only by board scores and other academic measures, but also by objective measurements of the mental health of their students and graduate physicians. This data, collected anonymously, ideally by medical student organizations and reported in the aggregate should be publicly available to prospective students.

This will not happen if we simply leave it up to our medical schools. They want to report inputs (we have X number of counselors available or we teach relaxation and coping techniques) but they don't want to objectively measure outcomes. It is time for those involved in medical education to consider innovative modification of the academic process combined with outcomes data to improve the mental health and wellbeing of physicians in training.

I have again filed HB 867, the "Show Me Compassionate Medical Education Act," in the Missouri House, this time for the 2016 session, and I intend to work to secure its passage. Thanks in no small measure to your untiring work on behalf of med students and physicians, there is a growing awareness in the medical community and in society that medical students and physicians are at increased risk of taking their own lives. My colleagues in the Missouri legislature understand that there is a problem that needs to be addressed in medical education. We can't bring back student doctor Kevin Dietl or Dr. Greg Miday, but we can act now to stop these tragedies. We don't want to lose one more physician-in-training to suicide.

Sincerely,
Keith
State Representative Dr. Keith J. Frederick
Missouri's 121st District

XIV

You Can Help

We're used to being on call for our patients.
I wonder what would happen if we were on call for each other.

49

Esther

November 20, 2014

Dear Pamela,

As a medical resident who has suffered with depression and suicidal thoughts for a large part of my career, I am so incredibly grateful that you are advocating for better understanding, more resources, and less stigma for doctors dealing with depression. I want to get involved. I am passionate about this topic, and I am disgusted by the lack of resources for medical students and residents going through training. I refuse to believe that medicine should be practiced by ruthless and egotistical psychopaths who think that mental illness is a sign of weakness. We are treating human beings and we are human beings. I want to help bring humanity back into this profession. How can I get involved at this level?

Esther

* * *

November 20, 2014

Dear Esther,

Thanks for writing to me. There are so many ways you can get involved.

1) Raise public awareness of physician suicide. Please share my article "Physician Suicide 101: Secrets, Lies & Solutions" [see Resources]. There's a huge lack of awareness and, sadly, a lot of denial among doctors. We can't solve a problem if nobody knows it exists!

2) Be kind to all medical students and doctors (even the mean ones). We need to change the culture of medicine. We each can do that now.

3) Implement the strategies I propose in the article. Learn and teach non-violent communication, for example. Start a peer support group. I have lots of other ideas too! Call me anytime 541-345-2437.

Pamela

50

Elizabeth

February 23, 2015

Pamela,

I lost another colleague and friend to suicide two weeks ago. As he was an anesthesiologist and I am an obstetrician, I saw him every day and had no clue that he was in such a state of despair. How can we recognize others in trouble?

Thanks,
Elizabeth

* * *

February 24, 2015

Elizabeth,

Suicide among physicians and medical students is unique when compared to the general population. I spoke recently with two retired police officers, parents of a physician friend. They've walked into numerous suicide scenes. They tell me that most people in the general population do not leave notes and usually have behavior changes that worry friends and family in the time leading up to their suicides.

Physicians typically are very high-functioning until their last breath. They're performing complex surgeries just hours before dying by suicide. Physicians also are very good at documenting and leaving notes. These suicide notes should be studied for common themes. Who is doing this? I'm analyzing every letter I receive and I strongly believe that nearly all of these suicides are preventable if we simply start taking appropriate action to remove the threats to doctors' lives. **The instructions are in their letters!**

If you encounter a suspicious death or suicide of a colleague, please don't sweep it under the rug. Hold a morbidity and mortality conference (as you would for a suspicious death in a patient) to investigate what it is that you and your medical institution can do to prevent the next tragedy. Suicide is preventable.

So how can we recognize those in trouble? Pay attention to even minor behavior changes and any and all complaints from physicians. A doctor who says, "I had a rough day" may actually be crying out for help. Befriend one another—especially male physicians. My informal collection of hundreds of completed suicide cases reveals that for every suicided female med student/physician, we lose seven males. Men do not generally ask for help. Anesthesiologists are high risk. Hug all male anesthesiologists!

We need a medical culture that supports our emotional health, that normalizes our need for comfort and non-punitive help when we're in pain. Until then, please reach out to each other. Maybe a buddy system. Don't allow doctors to isolate.

Pamela

51

Dan

March 13, 2015

Dear Pamela,

I'm going to tell you a personal story about a suicide that has haunted me for years. I worked as a clinic manager in town with a couple of doctors, Drs. Smith and Peterson. When our clinic hired Dr. Smith's wife, she told me to handle her husband with kid gloves. It was a mistake for me to have worked in this clinic. When I left I had an exit interview with both doctors. I was young and arrogant and told Dr. Smith to retire because his style of medicine was not good medicine. I left town and moved out of state. I later learned that Dr. Smith committed suicide. I was so crushed that I questioned everything I did after that. I carry a lot of guilt. You are the first person I have talked to about this.

Dan

* * *

June 2, 2015

Pamela,

I'm working at an internal medicine clinic in Washington and it's because of our conversation that I feel I have a depressed physician on my hands and I am addressing it as gently as I can. Thank you for your insights.

Dan

52

Gregory

April 23, 2014

Pamela,

I have been a physician for seventeen years now. I have what some would call a very successful career. I have been through two divorces in the past seven years. I had one close call with a suicide attempt six years ago and a truly attempted suicide eighteen months ago. I have not decided that I won't try it again. I want to say thank you for putting this information out.

Is there a way that we can change this? I have a good counselor, and I am on good meds. I just don't know how much more of my heart and soul I can prostitute to the powers that be anymore. These are more rhetorical questions. I just want to say thank you for doing this.

Gregory

* * *

April 23, 2014

Gregory,

Please come to my physician retreat next month. I'll waive the tuition. Do not sacrifice your beautiful life for our wounded profession. Please. Call me: 541-345-2437. I'm up now. I'm nocturnal. Impossible to disturb me.

Pamela

Addendum: Gregory came to the retreat (twice!) and is now helping other medical students and doctors heal. You can heal the healers too! Gregory is featured in "Our message of hope for medical students & doctors" [see Resources]. He's the big friendly guy you just want to hug at the beginning and end of the seven-minute video. If you want to help us help other healers heal, please contact me! I need help!

53

Varun

November 18, 2014

Dear Pamela,

You don't know how thankful I am to you for writing that article on physician suicide. I really wanted to hug you after reading it. I had a really rough day, 130 outpatients and sixty emergency admissions in a twelve-hour duty. I work as a final-year internal medicine resident in one of the busiest hospitals in India. I saw a part of myself in every page of your article. Just couldn't stop reading the article. It is 3:00 a.m. in the morning here and after a physically and mentally demanding day of work and studies, reading your article was the best thing today.

It takes me five hours by flight to reach my home from my hospital. I have my wife and six-month-old son (whom I've been with for fifteen days since his birth) at home. I work day in and out just to be with them once in three months. I don't see my colleagues smile, I hear my patients' misery every day. I smile and crack jokes even when I am sad so that I can bring some joy into my patients' sorrowful lives.

Today I saw this patient who died, married with a son, the only earning member of his family. His widow just wouldn't accept that he was dead. She kept talking to him. I just didn't know what to feel. I was numb for a minute thinking what if that was me. And the kid was my son . . .

I see deaths every day in ward. I don't know if you would believe me, but four deaths per day in a single ward of forty beds overcrowded to 125 patients admitted at a time. Two patients on a bed, two lying together on the floor. Poverty, misery, and pain all around. I have declared twelve patients dead in a day during one of my duties. I just don't feel death anymore, just don't feel human. My uncle died recently; I felt nothing deep inside—just some memories and that is it.

I write this mail hoping that the way I survive my day will help you in helping others.

I always wish my colleagues well and say hi when I see them in the morning. I say hi to everyone from my ward sweeper to the guard in the ward. I never eat alone and always make sure I share my food. I always smile whenever I talk to my patients. I hold their hands when I talk. Listen to music whenever possible. And every day whenever possible I talk to my wife, father, mother, and brother (all of them are doctors).

But still this profession demands too much from us. I have thought about giving up and suicide a thousand times—the misery is too much for me to see twelve people die in a day. The only thing that keeps me moving forward is my family and friends.

I appreciate what you are doing. It took me four hours to write this mail. It is seven in the morning. But your article was worth it. Thank you. Thanks a lot . . .

Dr. Varun

* * *

November 19, 2014

Dearest Varun,

Love from the USA to India & to you! Sending so much love to you, my brother!

XOX
Pamela

* * *

November 19, 2014

Pamela,

Thank you. Thanks a million from India and a lot of smiles for a beautiful mind. Have a nice day. I mean good-night. It should be night there.

Varun

* * *

November 26, 2014

Pamela,

Thank you! Thank you all for the support and love, for publishing my letter on your blog and for all the responses—the letters of support from USA.

Most of us here have adjusted to the situation. It is not lack of resources or manpower. The problem is inequality of their distribution in the society. I can see a Ferrari and Audi in the streets; I can see malls and supermarkets; I see luxury at a particular strata of society and poverty and misery in another. My society demands and forces these lifestyles on doctors. And funniest part is by forty you are bald with specs and a big tummy. Many patients here don't consider you as a doctor if you don't have all three of these. In life bad days aren't forever. I can wait for the better days. After all God has gifted me with an opportunity to wipe tears of many. To hold their hands and spread love. To see the sorrow in the eyes and replace it with hope. Thanks for your support. Lots of prayers and love from India.

With love,
Varun

* * *

November 29, 2014

Dear Varun,

I hear your suffering through your letter [on Pamela's blog]—and I hear the suffering of those you care for and I feel deep sadness, compassion, and sympathy. It sounds so very hard. That's awful.

One of the most powerful prayers I have learned from my medicine elders is, "May I never know how much I have helped somebody." When I first heard that I thought what a strange, backward-sounding thing to say! Now I understand it to protect me and the people I serve from enlarging my ego, that which causes separation, which is the opposite of healing. Despite the difficult and dark times, I choose to serve in the knowledge that I may be able to help, but I may never know how, or how much. I hold the door open for hope, movement, growth, healing, transformation—as they pass through invisible to me, visible only to those for whom I hold the door open.

When I need to know whether that works or how that is, I need only recall the small actions of others that were at the tipping point for me, that unbeknownst to them made all the difference in my life. The woman who spoke to me kindly at the public market on the day that I stood on the threshold of taking my own life. The one who encouraged me to finish my education. The one who stopped to see if I was okay when I crashed my bike and was nearly run over by a logging truck (the truck didn't stop). The man that smiled at me across the room and silently encouraged me to speak out in public for the voiceless ones, when I was afraid.

When I think of you far across the ocean at night, and all the miles of darkness between and around us, I picture your message that took so many hours to write, as a small light shining across the distance. I hope, as you read this, that you can picture a whole sea of little twinkling floating lights, a beautiful golden net of individual thoughtful, encouraging thoughts and well wishes for you, floating on the ocean, or on the air currents. From me. From us, your other selves. I am heartened by you, your enduring efforts, your vulnerability, your numbness. Your wholeness. And your calling out to Pamela and us in a way that affirms that between us all.

I am reminded of how instantly and effortlessly light can fill a vast space. I am learning to look to those things easily within my reach which can help make life easier for someone who may be far away and unable to make the changes I can by the simple act of flipping a light switch, of speaking out freely, of loving where I am. I simply echo from my experience, love never dies. Know that your smile is that light switch for many with whom you come into contact, and that the source of that light is clearly shining within your heart. Thank you for opening it to share with us. I see your light and it gives me hope and fortifies my resolve to keep doing my best for all the people. Like you.

Rachel

"I want to thank you for shining your light into the darkness, because if we all shine our lights together, there is no darkness to fear."

THE END . . . is just an illusion.

Conclusion

I never went looking for suicides. These suicides found me. I have many suicide letters. This book contains only a small sample. Amid the letters and calls from struggling doctors, I also receive heartbreaking letters from patients like this one:

"Dear Dr. Wible, I just got home from another insulting, degrading appointment with my doctor. I'm literally crying as I write to you. . ."

I called her. She shared her horror story. I shared mine. She never knew doctors could be suicidal. She never knew that she could be the victim in a cycle of abuse that began on day one of med school when her "insulting" doctor was still an idealistic student. How could she know that abused medical students become abused doctors who may one day abuse patients?

To all those who have been injured by our medical system, I am sorry. I am sorry that parents who had planned to attend their child's medical school graduation instead attend their child's funeral. I am so sorry that doctors wear forced smiles while living lives of silent desperation for fear of seeking help for their trauma. And I am so very, very sorry that patients receive the scraps we offer them as wounded healers. We all deserve better.

This cycle of health care abuse is a global phenomenon. Letters in this book are from Canada, Egypt, India, South Africa, UK, and the USA. There is no country in which medical students are immune from the effects of a traumatic medical education. There is no perfect health system in which doctors do not struggle to preserve their humanity and patients do not die for lack of care. There is no amount of money, no high-priced health plan that will guarantee that the doctor controlling your ventilator is not sleep-deprived or suicidal. We are all at risk.

So how do we stop the cycle of institutional abuse? Physician suicide hotlines *inside* our hospitals? Resilience training for our wiped-out doctors? Meditation classes for medical students? Advocacy centers for mistreated patients?

We must decide if our goal is to help victims cope with abuse or to end the abuse. I choose the latter. It's not costly or complicated to stop bullying, hazing, and abuse. It's been outlawed from elementary schools to fraternities and pretty much everywhere. Why not health care?

Medical culture and education must change. Yet cultures and institutions don't change because we ask them to change—even when it's in their self-interest. They change when they are forced to change. I favor the honor system. But what if those in charge are not behaving honorably? What if our medical system continues to blame, shame, and publicly humiliate its victims? What if that same system continues to deny, lie, look the other way, and—all too often—engage in a deliberate, active, ongoing cover-up of the facts about physician suicide? What can we do to stop this? I believe we can force change by simply shining a public spotlight on physician suicide.

Health care abuse is an assault on us all, and the cycle of abuse will be perpetuated—until someone stops it. That someone is you. So take action. Speak up when you witness bullying or abuse. If you feel mistreated as a patient, write a letter listing your complaints. Make positive suggestions when possible. If all else fails, boycott abusive health care systems. Tell your doctor you're no longer interested in supporting assembly-line medicine. Support ideal care for patients—and doctors.

Of course, some major institutional and legislative reforms are needed as well. Happily, we are starting to see a few proposals here and there—real steps toward curing our highly dysfunctional medical system. Some of those reforms are touched on in this book, such as the "Show Me Compassionate Medical Education Act," sponsored by Missouri State Representative Dr. Keith J. Frederick.

Ultimately, however, we will not be saved by laws and regulations alone. The factor that will make it possible for us to achieve these desperately needed changes is the light of compassion and truth that shines in each individual. That light is in this book. It blazes in the words of the doctors, patients, students, mothers, fathers, friends, colleagues, and fellow citizens whose letters are presented here.

We can heal each other. I know. In my darkest moments, patients have healed me. As my patient Rachel wrote in the final letter, "Love never dies." In my own journey to learn what leads to physician suicide and how we can prevent it, I know the truth of Rachel's words. I have seen that there is a love that is stronger than life, and even stronger than death. This is the love that will fuel the inevitable transformation of medicine. This is the love that will save us all.

On behalf of those we've lost and those who are barely hanging on, I thank you for spreading your love and shining your light into this world. We need you.

Acknowledgments

I am forever grateful to the courageous families who have allowed me to publish their children's suicide letters. To those who are struggling with suicidal thoughts, I thank you for permitting me to share your moments of deep despair with the world. Your words will forever offer clarity, validation, and healing for so many others. By witnessing your pain, I hope that I've helped you find strength and healing.

I thank all the dedicated people who spent their holiday season reading suicide letters: Marcus Webb, Betsy Robinson, Sydney Ashland, Karen Miday, Michele and John Dietl, Shelby Schneider, Keith Frederick, Jana Wolf Sussman, Ronae Jull, Victor Rozek, Kassy Daggett, Vicki DeHoff, William Smith, Sara Thurgood, Melissa Mason, Yvonne Whitelaw, Jill Zeiger, Laura Golson, Marianne Trevorrow, Steven Marks, Alison Alford, Michael Latteri, Janine Hantsch, Anna Gajewski, Tara Kruse, and K.G. Smith. You all are a very special crowd!

To my beautiful friend and director of photography, GeVe, I can never thank you enough. For years, you've documented my every move in my lectures, retreats, and private moments. You've uncovered this tragedy right alongside me. You've often shed more tears than anyone in the room (except maybe me) and carried suffering that is not yours to bear so that others may see, hear, and feel the truth of the medical students and doctors you have filmed and comforted. No doubt you have helped save countless lives.

Thanks to my powerhouse team I brought this book to life in record time. I wrote it in one week! Then edited it over the next three weeks. Finally, Kassy Daggett and I had the thing formatted, produced, and uploaded to Amazon in twenty-four hours.

People often ask me where I get the stamina to take on physician suicide. I was raised by a sarcastic, antisocial psychiatrist (I love you, Mom!) and an eccentric, obsessive compulsive pathologist. To survive my childhood, I had to be an expert in physician psychology. As a kid, I worked with Dad in the morgue. So I don't fear death. To my parents, Judith Wible and Theodore Krouse, I'm pretty damn sure I couldn't have done any of this without you!

Resources

Because this book addresses an international audience, I'm not listing country-specific hotlines. In addition, I only recommend resources that I have vetted or that have been useful to those who have contacted me. These resources have helped those in this book find their way back to life.

Publications

"Physician Suicide 101: Secrets, Lies & Solutions"
IdealMedicalCare.org/blog/physician-suicide-101-secrets-lies-solutions

"How to graduate medical school without killing yourself"
IdealMedicalCare.org/blog/how-to-graduate-medical-school-without-killing-yourself

Pamela Wible, M.D., blog at IdealMedicalCare.org/blog
See the categories "Medical Student Suicide" and "Physician Suicide"

Pet Goats & Pap Smears: 101 Medical Adventures to Open Your Heart & Mind
A book by Pamela Wible, M.D., that celebrates the joy of medicine

My Bright Shining Star: A Mother's True Story of Brilliance, Love & Suicide
A book by Rhonda Elkins about her daughter Kaitlyn (chapter 28)

Videos

TEDMED talk: "Why doctors kill themselves"
tedmed.com/talks/show?id=528918

TEDx talk: "How to get naked with your doctor"
youtube.com/watch?v=5cvHgGM-cRI

"Our message of hope for medical students & doctors"
IdealMedicalCare.org/blog/our-message-of-hope-for-medical-students-doctors

Medical Student & Physician Retreat

This retreat is open to anyone in health care who needs healing.
beahappydoctor.com (scholarships available)

Pamela Wible, M.D.

I welcome letters, emails, phone calls, and visitors :)
IdealMedicalCare.org/contact.php
P.O. Box 5225, Eugene, Oregon 97405
541-345-2437

If you are actively suicidal, please call a friend or a family member. Be with the people who love you. If you are unable to reach anyone who can be with you, please call the suicide hotline in your country or go to the nearest emergency room for help.

Cover Credits & Controversy

Design & production: Pamela Wible, Kassy Daggett
Photography & photo editing: GeVe, Michael Backus
Front cover suicide letter: Greg Miday

I've been absolutely fascinated by the controversy that my back cover has elicited among readers. I've been warned that I'm sabotaging myself with this author photo. For some, it's bizarre to see a doctor smiling in a bathtub on a suicide book. It's too weird and creepy because people often slit their wrists while taking a warm bath. It's just all wrong. Which is why it is right.

Greg Miday died in secrecy and shame by slitting his wrists and ankles in a bathtub. I'm bringing honesty and openness to his death and to a taboo topic that has been buried in darkness for far too long. From a hot tub. In the light of day. Smiling. Despite the fact that I treat sick patients all day and that I hear from suicidal doctors all the time, I am committed to living life joyfully with hope and optimism. My photo reflects that.

I've been advised that this cover could not possibly be comforting to anyone who has lost somebody to suicide. Then survivors of suicide attempts tell me they love the cover because it is reassuring and hopeful. I've been told the book cover succeeds in "comforting the disturbed and disturbing the comfortable."

I am a woman who elicits controversy, not because I enjoy controversy (although I do), but because I strive to stand in the truth. How I practice medicine has been controversial—from thriving in a solo practice where nobody is turned away for lack of money to being the voice of doctors who are disheartened, discouraged, depressed, and deceased.

Victims on front cover from left to right:
Bobby Bowling, Philip Henderson, Kevin Dietl,
Kaitlyn Elkins, Vincent Uybarreta, Greg Miday.

Rest in peace, sweet souls
(and keep in touch).